Endoscopy in the Era of Antibiotic Resistant Bacteria

Editor

JACQUES VAN DAM

GASTROINTESTINAL ENDOSCOPY CLINICS OF NORTH AMERICA

www.giendo.theclinics.com

Consulting Editor
CHARLES J. LIGHTDALE

October 2020 • Volume 30 • Number 4

ELSEVIER

1600 John F. Kennedy Boulevard • Suite 1800 • Philadelphia, Pennsylvania, 19103-2899

http://www.theclinics.com

GASTROINTESTINAL ENDOSCOPY CLINICS OF NORTH AMERICA Volume 30, Number 4
October 2020 ISSN 1052-5157, ISBN-13: 978-0-323-73386-1

Editor: Kerry Holland
Developmental Editor: Donald Mumford

Gastrointestinal Endoscopy Clinics of North America (ISSN 1052-5157) is published quarterly by Elsevier Inc., 360 Park Avenue South, New York, NY 10010-1710. Months of issue are January, April, July, and October. Business and Editorial Offices: 1600 John F. Kennedy Blvd., Suite 1800, Philadelphia, PA, 19103-2899. Periodicals postage paid at New York, NY and additional mailing offices. Subscription prices are $359.00 per year for US individuals, $655.00 per year for US institutions, $100.00 per year for US and Canadian students/residents, $399.00 per year for Canadian individuals, $774.00 per year for Canadian institutions, $476.00 per year for international individuals, $774.00 per year for international institutions, and $245.00 per year for international students/residents. To receive student/resident rate, orders must be accompanied by name of affiliated institution, date of term, and the *signature* of program/residency coordinator on institution letterhead. Orders will be billed at individual rate until proof of status is received. Foreign air speed delivery is included in all *Clinics* subscription prices. All prices are subject to change without notice. **POSTMASTER:** Send address change to *Gastrointestinal Endoscopy Clinics of North America*, Elsevier Health Sciences Division, Subscription Customer Service, 3251 Riverport Lane, Maryland Heights, MO 63043. **Customer Service: 1-800-654-2452 (US). From outside the United States, call 1-314-447-8871. Fax: 1-314-447-8029. E-mail: JournalsCustomerService-usa@elsevier.com (for print support) or JournalsOnlineSupport-usa@elsevier.com (for online support).**

Reprints. For copies of 100 or more, of articles in this publication, please contact the Commercial Reprints Department, Elsevier Inc., 360 Park Avenue South, New York, NY 10010-1710. Tel. 212-633-3874; Fax: 212 633-3820; E-mail: reprints@elsevier.com.

Gastrointestinal Endoscopy Clinics of North America is covered in *Excerpta Medica, MEDLINE/PubMed (Index Medicus), and MEDLINE/MEDLARS.*

Contributors

CONSULTING EDITOR

CHARLES J. LIGHTDALE, MD
Professor of Medicine, Division of Digestive and Liver Diseases, Columbia University Medical Center, New York, New York, USA

EDITOR

JACQUES VAN DAM, MD, PhD
Professor of Medicine, (Clinical Scholar), Keck School of Medicine, University of Southern California, Los Angeles, California, USA

AUTHORS

MICHELLE J. ALFA, PhD, FCCM
Department of Medical Microbiology, University of Manitoba, Winnipeg, Manitoba, Canada

MATTHEW J. ARDUINO, DrPH
Division of Healthcare Quality Promotion, Centers for Disease Control and Prevention, Atlanta, Georgia, USA

SUBHAS BANERJEE, MD
Professor of Medicine, Division of Gastroenterology and Hepatology, Stanford University School of Medicine, Stanford, California, USA

MONIQUE T. BARAKAT, MD, PhD
Assistant Professor of Medicine and Pediatrics, Divisions of Adult and Pediatric Gastroenterology and Hepatology, Stanford University School of Medicine, Stanford, California, USA

ISAAC BENOWITZ, MD
Division of Healthcare Quality Promotion, Centers for Disease Control and Prevention, Atlanta, Georgia, USA

TYLER M. BERZIN, MD, FASGE
Assistant Professor of Medicine, Division of Gastroenterology, Center for Advanced Endoscopy, Beth Israel Deaconess Medical Center, Harvard Medical School, Boston, Massachusetts, USA

BRIAN P. H. CHAN, MD, FRCPC
Division of Gastroenterology, Center for Advanced Endoscopy, Beth Israel Deaconess Medical Center, Harvard Medical School, Boston, Massachusetts, USA

STEPHANIE COLE, PhD
United States Food and Drug Administration, Office of Medical Products and Tobacco, Center for Devices and Radiological Health, Office of Health Technology 3, Silver Spring, Maryland, USA

JIAN CONNELL, DNP, MSN, CPN
United States Food and Drug Administration, Office of Medical Products and Tobacco, Center for Devices and Radiological Health, Office of Health Technology 3, Silver Spring, Maryland, USA

ANNABELLE de St. MAURICE, MD, MPH
Assistant Professor Pediatric Infectious Diseases, Co-Infection Prevention Officer UCLA Health, Department of Pediatrics, David Geffen School of Medicine at UCLA, UCLA Clinical Epidemiology and Infection Prevention, Los Angeles, California, USA

JANA K. DICKTER, MD
Associate Clinical Professor, Division of Infectious Diseases, City of Hope, Duarte, California, USA

LAUREN EPSTEIN, MD
Division of Healthcare Quality Promotion, Centers for Disease Control and Prevention, Atlanta, Georgia, USA

ANN FERRITER
United States Food and Drug Administration, Office of Medical Products and Tobacco, Center for Devices and Radiological Health, Office of Health Technology 3, Silver Spring, Maryland, USA

SHANIL P. HAUGEN, PhD
United States Food and Drug Administration, Office of Medical Products and Tobacco, Center for Devices and Radiological Health, Office of Health Technology 3, Silver Spring, Maryland, USA

JENNIFER T. HIGA, MD
Division of Gastroenterology, Fox Chase Cancer Center, Philadelphia, Pennsylvania, USA

KARL K. KWOK, MD
Division of Gastroenterology, Southern California Kaiser Permanente Medical Group, Los Angeles, California, USA

JIA-YIA LIU, MD
Assistant Clinical Professor, Department of Medicine, Loma Linda University, Loma Linda, California, USA; President and Director, American Medical Physicians and Surgeons Advancement Alliance, Pasadena, California, USA; Attending Physician, Division of Infectious Diseases, Cedars-Sinai Medical Center, Los Angeles, California, USA

QUIN Y. LIU, MD
Assistant Clinical Professor of Pediatrics and Medicine, Cedars-Sinai Medical Center/ David Geffen School of Medicine at UCLA, Department of Medicine and Pediatrics, Digestive Disease Center, Los Angeles, California, USA

NEIL B. MARYA, MD
Vatche and Tamar Manoukian Division of Digestive Diseases, David Geffen School of Medicine at UCLA, Los Angeles, California, USA

LAUREN J. MIN, PhD
United States Food and Drug Administration, Office of Medical Products and Tobacco, Center for Devices and Radiological Health, Office of Health Technology 3, Silver Spring, Maryland, USA

LINDSAY MORRISON, MD
Fellow, Division of Infectious Disease, McGaw Medical Center, Northwestern University Feinberg School of Medicine, Chicago, Illinois, USA

HEATHER A. MOULTON-MEISSNER, PhD
Division of Healthcare Quality Promotion, Centers for Disease Control and Prevention, Atlanta, Georgia, USA

RAMAN V. MUTHUSAMY, MD, MAS, AGAF, FASGE, FACG
Medical Director of Endoscopy, Professor of Clinical Medicine, Vatche and Tamar Manoukian Division of Digestive Diseases, David Geffen School of Medicine at UCLA, Los Angeles, California, USA

ANDREW S. ROSS, MD
Division of Gastroenterology, Virginia Mason Medical Center, Seattle, Washington, USA

ZACHARY A. RUBIN, MD
Medical Epidemiologist Chief, Healthcare Outreach Unit, Acute Communicable Disease Control, Los Angeles County Department of Public Health, Los Angeles, California, USA

GRAHAM M. SNYDER, MD, SM
Department of Infection Control and Hospital Epidemiology, University of Pittsburgh Medical Center, Division of Infectious Diseases, University of Pittsburgh School of Medicine, Pittsburgh, Pennsylvania, USA

DAVID S. VITALE, MD
Assistant Professor of Pediatrics, Division of Gastroenterology, Hepatology and Nutrition, Department of Pediatrics, Cincinnati Children's Hospital Medical Center, University of Cincinnati College of Medicine, Cincinnati, Ohio, USA

HANNIEBEY D. WIYOR, PhD, RAC
United States Food and Drug Administration, Office of Medical Products and Tobacco, Center for Devices and Radiological Health, Office of Health Technology 3, Silver Spring, Maryland, USA

TERESA R. ZEMBOWER, MD, MPH
Associate Professor of Medicine (Infectious Disease) and Pathology, Northwestern University Feinberg School of Medicine, Chicago, Illinois, USA

Contents

Pathogen contamination of endoscopes depends on pathogen factors, surface factors, and environmental conditions. The most common pathogens associated with transmission and infections associated with gastrointestinal endoscope contamination are Klebsiella pneumoniae, Escherichia coli, and Pseudomonas aeruginosa. Biofilm production together with disruption to device surfaces play an outsized role in the risk of contamination. Sampling schemes are limited by these factors, and further developments are needed to improve the accuracy of sampling.

Antimicrobial resistance is developing rapidly and threatens to outstrip the rate at which new antimicrobials are introduced. Genetic recombination allows bacteria to rapidly disseminate genes encoding for antimicrobial resistance within and across species. Antimicrobial use creates a selective evolutionary pressure, which leads to further resistance. Antimicrobial stewardship, best use, and infection prevention are the most effective ways to slow the spread and development of antimicrobial resistance.

In the United States, healthcare acquired infections (HAIs) or nosocomial infections are the sixth leading cause of death. This article reviews the history, prevalence, economic costs, morbidity and mortality, and risk factors associated with HAIs. Types of infections described include bacterial, fungal, viral, and multidrug resistant infections that contribute to the most common causes of HAIs, which include catheter- associated urinary tract infections, hospital-acquired pneumonias, bloodstream infections, and surgical site infections. Most nosocomial infections are preventable and monitoring and prevention strategies are described.

factors all contribute to contamination of patient-ready endoscopes that may contribute to transmission of microorganisms resulting in infection and/or colonization. This article reviews monitoring as part of a quality management system that includes manual cleaning, dry storage, and culture to detect endoscope contamination. The published data for rapid tests that detect organic residuals and adenosine triphosphate to monitor manual cleaning are reviewed.

In addition to technological advancements, engagement and collaboration among the wider community of stakeholders will be beneficial toward reducing the risk of infection from reprocessed duodenoscopes. Such a community can raise awareness of the importance of duodenoscope cleaning, work to improve reprocessing training, identify the most pressing unanswered questions that merit further research, and develop tools that can be used by health care facilities to improve the quality of reprocessing at their sites. The Food and Drug Administration looks forward to working with the community to further reduce the risk of infections from reprocessed duodenoscopes.

Flexible endoscopes require cleaning, high-level disinfection, and sterilization between each patient use to reduce risk of transmitting pathogens. Public health investigations have identified concerns, including endoscope damage, mishandling, and reprocessing deficiencies, placing patients at risk for transmission of bacterial, viral, and other pathogens. Findings from outbreak investigations and other studies have led to innovations in endoscope design, use, and reprocessing, yet infection risks related to contaminated or damaged endoscopes remain. Strict adherence to infection control guidelines and manufacturer instructions for use, utilization of supplemental guidance, and training and oversight of reprocessing personnel, reduce risk of pathogen transmission by flexible endoscopes.

Transmission of pathogens during endoscopy and subsequent outbreak investigations generated by potential nosocomial transmissions have become a major concern for gastroenterologists. These investigations have resulted in significant media coverage for individual institutions and can cause massive disruption to the institution if not handled well. Gastroenterologists should have a central role in investigation of these outbreaks and management of the communications and patient notification that is required. This article summarizes important aspects of outbreak

GASTROINTESTINAL ENDOSCOPY CLINICS OF NORTH AMERICA

RELATED CLINICS SERIES

Gastroenterology Clinics
(www.gastro.theclinics.com)
Clinics in Liver Disease
(www.liver.theclinics.com)

THE CLINICS ARE AVAILABLE ONLINE!
Access your subscription at:
www.theclinics.com

GASTROINTESTINAL ENDOSCOPY CLINICS
OF NORTH AMERICA

FORTHCOMING ISSUES

January 2021
Advances in Barrett's Esophagus
Sachin Wani, Editor

April 2021
Video Capsule Endoscopy
David Cave, Editor

July 2021
Gastric Cancer
Chin Hur, Editor

RECENT ISSUES

July 2020
Colorectal Cancer Screening
Douglas K. Rex, Editor

April 2020
Management of GERD: Looking into 2020
Vision
Kenneth J. Chang, Editor

January 2020
Endoscopic Closure Techniques: Endoscopic
Closing Over-The-Scope (OTS) and
Endoscopic Suturing
Roy Soetikno and Tonya Kaltenbach,
Editors

RELATED CLINICS SERIES

Gastroenterology Clinics
(www.gastro.theclinics.com)
Clinics in Liver Disease
(www.liver.theclinics.com)

THE CLINICS ARE AVAILABLE ONLINE!
Access your subscription at:
www.theclinics.com

Foreword

Endoscopes and Antibiotic-Resistant Bacteria: Controlling the Risk

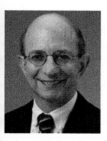

Charles J. Lightdale, MD
Consulting Editor

Threats to highly valuable systems abound in modern society. Think of airplanes for example. Changes are made, and innovations are developed, resulting in improved safety, only to be challenged by new risks. In the history of medicine, there have been many instances where inadvertent transmission of infection by physicians was identified, and corrective measures were taken. In modern times, antibiotic-resistant bacteria are among the latest microscopic terrorists. For interventional gastrointestinal endoscopists, the most prized instruments are duodenoscopes used mostly for endoscopic retrograde cholangiopancreatography. These instruments have certainly brought great benefit, avoiding costly and painful operations, and saving the lives of many patients. That these same duodenoscopes have transmitted often lethal antibiotic-resistant organisms to patients in localized outbreaks is now well documented. Why the duodenoscopes (and possibly linear ultrasound endoscopes) have this problem as opposed to other endoscopes is almost certainly that they have an elevator mechanism in the working channel for precise manipulation of instruments passed through the channel. These tiny mechanisms are difficult to clean and may allow biofilms to accumulate. The instruments are too delicate to sterilize. The response to this threat has been a more rigorous application and modification of the high-level disinfection procedures used for all endoscopes, and the introduction of regular surveillance of endoscopes by microbiology and infectious disease control. These changes seem to be working, but more time is needed to be certain. Meanwhile, transparency in informed consent with patients about the risks of infection particularly from duodenoscopes is essential. New instrument designs, including disposable elevators in the duodenoscope tip, and even disposable duodenoscopes are being tested. Whether any of these instruments will be as effective as the current scopes is a critical question.

Gastrointest Endoscopy Clin N Am 30 (2020) xiii–xiv
https://doi.org/10.1016/j.giec.2020.07.001
1052-5157/20/© 2020 Published by Elsevier Inc.

giendo.theclinics.com

I am very grateful to Dr Jacques Van Dam, the Editor for this issue of the *Gastrointestinal Endoscopy Clinics of North America* devoted to "Endoscopy in the Era of Antibiotic Resistant Bacteria." Dr Van Dam is a renowned thought-leader in gastrointestinal endoscopy, and he has selected expert authors and topics on antibiotic-resistant bacteria and endoscopes as potential vectors. There are several articles analyzing recent hospital outbreaks, on endoscope reprocessing, and comparing guidelines and quality recommendations. Key articles are included from the Food and Drug Administration and the Centers for Disease Control and Prevention. This thoroughly important issue of the *Gastrointestinal Endoscopy Clinics of North America* will surely be of interest to all gastrointestinal endoscopists.

Charles J. Lightdale, MD
Department of Medicine
Columbia University Medical Center
161 Fort Washington Avenue
New York, NY 10032, USA

E-mail address:
CJL18@columbia.edu

Preface

Gastrointestinal Endoscopy in the Era of Antibiotic Resistant Bacteria

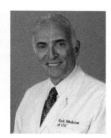

Jacques Van Dam, MD, PhD
Editor

What happened? How could it all go so terribly wrong? Where do we go from here?

For those of us who do endoscopic retrograde cholangiopancreatography, or for that matter interventional endoscopic ultrasonography (EUS), the last thing we ever want to do is harm a patient as a result of one of our procedures. We know these endoscopic tools to be essential in modern medical practice, offering a diagnosis or therapeutic intervention in many cases for our sickest patients. We think we understand the risks of our procedures, including the risk of infection. But after decades of apparently safe and successful advanced endoscopy, we have sidestepped into a problem with, in far too many instances, lethal consequences.

Is it really a lack of responsible antimicrobial stewardship that has led to the evolution of otherwise manageable bacteria into lethal, antibiotic-resistant pathogens? Or is it that our endoscopes are harboring a flawed technology? A technology that on the one hand enables us to intervene in ways that previous generations of physicians and surgeons would have thought miraculous but on the other hand creates hidden sanctuaries for bacteria to escape detection and elimination. Or is it our methods for cleaning and reprocessing our instruments in many instances without the proper safeguards and quality controls?

For those of us who have not experienced an outbreak through either luck or vigilance, let's see if we can learn something from those who have. I'd like to extend my sincere gratitude to those authors who have, by necessity, become experts in this area, for giving so freely of their time and expertise. I would especially like to thank those who have experienced firsthand what it is like to come to the realization that your center has experienced an outbreak and that you are at or near its core. Thank you for so generously sharing what you have learned so that we may benefit. I am

Gastrointest Endoscopy Clin N Am 30 (2020) xv–xvi
https://doi.org/10.1016/j.giec.2020.07.002
1052-5157/20/© 2020 Published by Elsevier Inc.

grateful to the infectious disease experts and epidemiologists who contribute to our understanding of the pathogens involved in the outbreaks and their modes of transmission. And I am most grateful to those from our nation's regulatory agencies, the Food and Drug Administration and the Centers for Disease Control and Prevention. Your offices are in the midst of trying to both resolve what happened and create, as much as possible, an evidenced-based response in an effort to protect the public. As endoscopists, we share in this endeavor and hope that together we can arrive at a sustainable solution.

Jacques Van Dam, MD, PhD
Keck School of Medicine
University of Southern California
1510 San Pablo Street, Suite 322R
Los Angeles, CA 90033, USA

E-mail address:
jvandam@usc.edu

Introduction to Transmission of Infection

Potential Agents Transmitted by Endoscopy

Graham M. Snyder, MD, SM[a,b,*]

KEYWORDS

- Environmental contamination • Medical devices • Fomites • Culture surveillance
- Endoscope sampling

KEY POINTS

- A diverse group of pathogens may contaminate endoscopes, but human endogenous bacterial flora are most commonly identified.
- Pathogen persistence on environmental surfaces is determined by the pathogen, the surface, and the environmental conditions.
- Variability and limitations in the methods used to recover pathogens from endoscope surfaces diminishes the reliability and validity of sampling programs.

INTRODUCTION

Acquiring an infection has always been a risk associated with receiving care in organized institutions, and the development of infection control programs in the mid to late twentieth century has abated but not eliminated this risk.[1] Many infections are due to the endogenous flora that comprise the human microbiome. The use of a foreign body as an indwelling medical device potentiates the risk for infection owing to endogenous flora (or rarely, owing to pathogens contaminating a purportedly sterile device); this risk associated with medical devices remains despite decades of investigation into the nature of device surfaces and the promise of pathogen-inhibiting technology.[2] Our environment has a microbiome of its own, and no surface in the health care environment can be guaranteed sterile. The environment serves as both reservoir and vehicle for transmission.[3]

The endoscope, particularly the gastrointestinal endoscope, has characteristics of risks associated with both a medical device and the environment. It is a multiuse device that transits and is a part of the health care environment. It is also a device with

[a] Department of Infection Control and Hospital Epidemiology, University of Pittsburgh Medical Center, Pittsburgh, PA, USA; [b] Division of Infectious Diseases, University of Pittsburgh School of Medicine, Pittsburgh, PA, USA
* 3601 5th Avenue, Falk Medical Building, Suite 150, Pittsburgh, PA 15213.
E-mail address: snydergm3@upmc.edu

Gastrointest Endoscopy Clin N Am 30 (2020) 611–618
https://doi.org/10.1016/j.giec.2020.05.001
giendo.theclinics.com

direct exposure to the prolific and diverse human intestinal microbiome—in an area often devoid of medical devices—and which is used in a way that provides a mucosal barrier-disruptive opportunity that can and does lead to invasive infections.[4]

This article seeks to put in context pathogen contamination of endoscopes and therefore the subsequent risk for transmission and infections. The article reviews the spectrum of pathogens potentially causing endoscope contamination, discusses the determinants of pathogen persistence on fomites, and previews challenges in recovering pathogens from surfaces.

THE SPECTRUM OF PATHOGENS POTENTIALLY CAUSING ENDOSCOPE CONTAMINATION

Pathogen contamination of endoscopes depends on pathogen factors, surface factors, and environmental conditions. A discussion of nosocomial infections can be found in (Jia-Yia Liu and Jana K. Dickter's article, "Nosocomial Infections – a History of Hospital-Acquired Infections," in this issue) and design characteristics of gastrointestinal endoscopes that predispose to contamination and transmission are discussed in (Jennifer T. Higa and Andrew S. Ross's article, "Duodenoscope as a Vector for Transmission," in this issue). Publications describing outbreaks associated with device contamination and routine culture surveillance provide insights into the pathogens that can and do cause endoscope contamination.

Bacterial, mycobacterial, viral, and fungal pathogens have all been described to contaminate endoscopes. In a review published in 2013, Kovaleva and colleagues[5] cataloged pathogens that have been demonstrated to be transmitted by flexible endoscope: systemic pathogens including *Pseudomonas aeruginosa* and *Serratia marcescens*, enteric bacterial pathogens such as *Helicobacter pylori* and *Salmonella* sp., spore-forming bacteria including *Clostridium difficile*, nontuberculous mycobacteria (and *Mycobacterium tuberculosis* associated with bronchoscopes), viral bloodborne pathogens including hepatitis B virus and hepatitis C virus (but to date, not human immunodeficiency virus), and parasites. Transmission of fungal pathogens by gastrointestinal endoscopes have not been previously described with the exception of 2 descriptions of *Trichosporon* sp. transmission,[5,6] but there is reason to believe that at least *Candida sp.* have the potential to be associated with transmission and infection, in part because surveillance studies have demonstrated yeast pathogens contaminating gastrointestinal endoscopes.[7,8]

More recent publications have demonstrated a distribution of transmitted (or putatively transmitted) pathogens heavily favoring *Enterobacteriaceae*, notably with the emergence in the last decade of publications describing duodenoscope-associated outbreaks with multidrug-resistant pathogens. Outbreaks have been associated with *K pneumoniae*,[9–17] *E coli*,[18–22] *P aeruginosa*,[23–26] and *Salmonella enteritidis*,[27] predominantly associated with a carbapenem-resistant phenotype with varied genetic mechanisms of resistance.[28]

This predilection for contamination and transmission with gram-negative bacilli has also been demonstrated in studies reporting contamination identified during routine culture surveillance. The breadth of pathogens in these studies also includes skin and environmental flora, however. Although systematic evaluations of duodenoscope contamination outside the outbreak setting have demonstrated contamination rates with pathogenic bacteria of 0% to 2%,[19,29–31] contamination with any bacteria is higher and described in the 5% to 25% range.[8,19,29,30,32,33]

Few studies have speciated all micro-organisms identified, but a recent study by Rauwers and colleagues[8] that included 73 Dutch facilities were 155 duodenoscopes from 3 manufacturers were sampled from between 1 and 7 sampling sites for a total of 745 samples. Data from 150 sampled duodenoscopes provides detailed nonregulatory published data of duodenoscope "flora": gastrointestinal flora (of any colony-forming unit [CFU] count) included unspeciated yeasts (7 duodenoscopes), *K pneumoniae*, *E coli*, and *P aeruginosa* (4, 2, and 1 duodenoscopes, respectively), *Enterobacter cloacae* (3), *Klebsiella oxytoca* (2), and gram-positive cocci (*Enterococcus faecium*, *Enterococcus faecalis*, and *Staphylococcus aureus* in 1 duodenoscope each). The authors also described 9 different oral flora genus or species of any CFU count (≤4 duodenoscopes each, predominantly *Moraxella* spp. and *Streptococcus* spp.), 10 different skin flora genus or species with 20 or more CFU growth (≤4 duodenoscopes each, predominantly non–*S aureus* staphylococci), and 10 different waterborne flora genus or species with 20 or more CFU growth (≤3 duodenoscopes each, including non–*P aeruginosa* pseudomonads, *Stenotrophomonas maltophilia*, and *Acinetobacter* spp.).[8] Other studies describing bacterial genera and species identified a similar complement of organisms from approximately 2 dozen positive samples each.[19,29] Last, the US Food and Drug Administration–mandated postmarketing surveillance studies are underway and will provide information on the pathogens contaminating duodenoscopes using the sampling method validated by the US Food and Drug Administration, the Centers for Disease Control and Prevention, and the American Society for Microbiology.[34] Preliminary data show contamination rates of up to 3.6% for low concern organisms (>100 CFU) and 5.4% of high concern organisms.[35]

There is marked difference between the varied bacterial species identified to contaminate endoscopes—particularly duodenoscopes for which the most data are available—and the relatively few species described in outbreaks. This difference is likely accounted for by the presence of pathogen factors that support persistence in the environment with or without the presence of virulence factors that lead to invasive infection.

DETERMINANTS OF PATHOGEN PERSISTENCE ON FOMITES

Combined with the virulence factors and antimicrobial resistance mechanisms (see Lindsay Morrison and Teresa R. Zembower's article, "Antimicrobial Resistance," in this issue) that contribute to significance of infections they cause, bacterial pathogens have various intrinsic mechanisms to promote survivability in the environment and on fomites. These factors interplay with characteristics of the surface and environmental conditions to produce the potential for endoscope contamination. The specific design characteristics of endoscopes that may lead to contamination and therefore pathogen transmission is reviewed in (Jennifer T. Higa and Andrew S. Ross's article, "Duodenoscope as a Vector for Transmission," in this issue).

The relationship between bacteria, surface material, and environmental conditions (such as in vitro vs in vivo conditions) are complicated and all affect the likelihood of persistent viable pathogens remaining on endoscopes. For example, characteristics of different bacteria (genus, species, gene carriage and gene expression) may result in different surface adhesion characteristics; for a specific strain, adhesion characteristics may not be the same for all material types; and the environment may affect pathogen characteristics such as biofilm formation.[2]

Accordingly, it is not surprising that studies of environmental survival of human pathogens show variability, including over orders of magnitude in some cases.[3,36,37] In a 2006 systematic review of nosocomial pathogen persistence on dry inanimate surfaces, *Klebsiella* spp., *E coli*, and *P aeruginosa* persistence ranged from 2 hours to more than 30 months, 1.5 hours to 16 months, and 6 hours to 16 months, respectively.[36] As outlined in this review, viruses have a generally shorter environmental persistence than bacteria and this factor may be important in the predilection of bacterial over viral pathogen transmission by contaminated endoscope. (Reproduction outside the host and pathogen frequency and density in the gastrointestinal tract may certainly be stronger explanations.)

Pathogen-intrinsic factors strongly influence the endoscope "flora" and therefore subsequent device-associated transmission and patient infection. *K pneumoniae*, for example, has multiple virulence factors that permit environmental persistence including fimbriae and capsular polysaccharides.[38,39] Fimbriae are a class of virulence factors that serve as adhesive structures, expressed in nearly all *K pneumoniae* isolates as well as other *Enterobacteriaceae*. Type 1 and type 3 fimbriae play multiple roles for the pathogen including expression in biofilms and adherence to abiotic surfaces.[38] Capsular polysaccharides also contribute to the virulence of the pathogen and play an important role in environmental persistence including the development of biofilms, which allow survival despite adverse environmental conditions.[38,39] An understanding of pathogen-intrinsic factors may aid in the development of interventions that reduce the risk of endoscope contamination.[40]

Surface characteristics, including device material and surface texture, also influence bacterial adherence.[2] The use of resin polymer coatings and steel may have properties that confer susceptibility to bacterial growth and persistence.[41] Furthermore, irregular surfaces from abrasion, erosion, and aging are highly likely to contribute to endoscope contamination; studies have shown the presence of biofilm, particularly in relation to disrupted surfaces, in the setting of endoscope contamination and pathogen transmission.[7,25,42]

Last, environmental conditions play a role in the contamination of duodenoscopes. Moisture is a factor that has been associated with growth and can be controlled by reprocessing methods.[43,44] Similarly, residual bioburden may allow for the continued growth of bacterial pathogens. Although the biofilm may limit the effectiveness of disinfectant and sterilant compounds, overt resistance is unlikely to play a significant role in endoscope contamination; there is 1 report of a glutaraldehyde-resistant *P aeruginosa* and resistance to aldehyde-based disinfectants is more prominently a feature of mycobacteria, which remain susceptible to other agents.[45]

What can be done to decrease or eliminate determinants of pathogen persistence on endoscope surfaces? The most practical approaches include single-use devices, modification to endoscope design, and/or fastidious and enhanced methods of endoscope reprocessing (see Jennifer T. Higa and Andrew S. Ross's article, "Duodenoscope as a Vector for Transmission," in this issue and Neil B. Marya and V. Raman Muthusamy's article, "Methods For Endoscope Reprocessing," in this issue). In the absence of changes to the endoscope or reprocessing, unconventional and perhaps controversial solutions may be required, such as the incorporation of antimicrobial surfaces[46,47] or the use of bacterial interference.[48,49]

CHALLENGES IN THE RECOVERY OF PATHOGENS FROM ENDOSCOPE SURFACES

These factors all conspire to limit the ability to recover pathogens from endoscopes, and the current recommended method for sampling endoscopes comes with the caveat that it "cannot be used to certify that an endoscope is sterile."[34] Indeed, there is no established gold standard for demonstrating microbial contamination of an endoscope, and there likely exists a reporting bias in studies of outbreaks and endoscope contamination—the methods used to identify microbes in part define the microbes that are identified.

With this in mind, the methods used to sample endoscopes may be improved by onsidering the potential reasons for persistent contamination. For example, several tudies suggest that sampling of the channel with using a brush or pull-through ponge with a fluid flush has a greater yield than a fluid flush alone, an effect likely elated to mechanical disruption of biofilm.[50,51] Similarly, a flocked swab rather than brush and the addition of fluid turbidity (by pipetting) to a brush increased the micro-ial yield from sampling of the duodenoscope elevator, again likely owing to biofilm isruption.[50–52] Further investigations including the use of sonication and biofilm-isrupting agents may improve the sensitivity of sampling methods to detect duode-oscope contamination.

Studies investigating methods for endoscope sampling and the current recommen-ed protocol for duodenoscope sampling all have laboratory cultivation techniques ailored toward bacterial pathogens. The association of mycobacterial and fungal in-ections associated with duodenoscope contamination may therefore go unde-ected.[53,54] Advanced molecular methods may in the future serve as a mechanism o identify more diverse contaminating pathogens with greater sensitivity, and with a horter turnaround time. In a singular study of multiplex real-time polymerase chain re-ction testing targeting bacterial genes, sensitivity and specificity were both 98% to letect contaminated and reprocessed colonoscopes.[55] Validation of this method vould be required, including against cultures from reprocessed duodenoscopes tar-eting bacterial, mycobacterial, and fungal pathogens.

UMMARY

tudies have demonstrated persistent endoscope contamination of endoscopes lespite appropriate reprocessing techniques. The risk of endoscope contamination nd therefore transmission of pathogen will likely remain given the intrinsic nature of ne exposure to endogenous flora with the ability to form biofilms and the surface char-cteristics of the endoscopes themselves. Identifying potential pathogens beyond the nost commonly identified bacteria—*K pneumoniae*, *E coli*, and *P aeruginosa*—will equire changes to sampling techniques.

ISCLOSURE

he author reports no commercial or financial conflicts of interest.

EFERENCES

1. Dixon RE, Centers for Disease Control and Prevention. Control of health-care-associated infections, 1961-2011. MMWR Suppl 2011;60(4):58–63.

2. Darouiche RO. Device-associated infections: a macroproblem that starts with mi-croadherence. Clin Infect Dis 2001;33(9):1567–72.

3. Suleyman G, Alangaden G, Bardossy AC. The role of environmental contamina-tion in the transmission of nosocomial pathogens and healthcare-associated in-fections. Curr Infect Dis Rep 2018;20(6):12.

4. Schlaeffer F, Riesenberg K, Mikolich D, et al. Serious bacterial infections after endoscopic procedures. Arch Intern Med 1996;156(5):572–4.

5. Kovaleva J, Peters FT, van der Mei HC, et al. Transmission of infection by flexible gastrointestinal endoscopy and bronchoscopy. Clin Microbiol Rev 2013;26(2):231–54.

6. ASGE Quality Assurance in Endoscopy Committee, Calderwood AH, Day LW, et al. ASGE guideline for infection control during GI endoscopy. Gastrointest Endosc 2018;87(5):1167–79.
7. Buss AJ, Been MH, Borgers RP, et al. Endoscope disinfection and its pitfalls requirement for retrograde surveillance cultures. Endoscopy 2008;40(4):327–32.
8. Rauwers AW, Voor In 't Holt AF, Buijs JG, et al. High prevalence rate of digestive tract bacteria in duodenoscopes: a nationwide study. Gut 2018;67(9):1637–45.
9. Aumeran C, Poincloux L, Souweine B, et al. Multidrug-resistant Klebsiella pneumoniae outbreak after endoscopic retrograde cholangiopancreatography. Endoscopy 2010;42(11):895–9.
10. Carbonne A, Thiolet JM, Fournier S, et al. Control of a multi-hospital outbreak of KPC-producing Klebsiella pneumoniae type 2 in France, September to October 2009. Euro Surveill 2010;15(48).
11. Alrabaa SF, Nguyen P, Sanderson R, et al. Early identification and control of carbapenemase-producing Klebsiella pneumoniae, originating from contaminated endoscopic equipment. Am J Infect Control 2013;41(6):562–4.
12. Gastmeier P, Vonberg RP. Klebsiella spp. in endoscopy-associated infections: we may only be seeing the tip of the iceberg. Infection 2014;42(1):15–21.
13. Kola A, Piening B, Pape UF, et al. An outbreak of carbapenem-resistant OXA-48-producing Klebsiella pneumonia associated to duodenoscopy. Antimicrob Resist Infect Control 2015;4:8.
14. Marsh JW, Krauland MG, Nelson JS, et al. Genomic Epidemiology of an Endoscope-Associated Outbreak of Klebsiella pneumoniae Carbapenemase (KPC)-Producing K. pneumoniae. PLoS One 2015;10(12):e0144310.
15. Humphries RM, Yang S, Kim S, et al. Duodenoscope-related outbreak of carbapenem-resistant klebsiella pneumoniae identified using advanced molecular diagnostics. Clin Infect Dis 2017;65(7):1159–66.
16. Bourigault C, Le Gallou F, Bodet N, et al. Duodenoscopy: an amplifier of cross-transmission during a carbapenemase-producing Enterobacteriaceae outbreak in a gastroenterology pathway. J Hosp Infect 2018;99(4):422–6.
17. Rauwers AW, Troelstra A, Fluit AC, et al. Independent root-cause analysis of contributing factors, including dismantling of 2 duodenoscopes, to investigate an outbreak of multidrug-resistant Klebsiella pneumoniae. Gastrointest Endosc 2019;90(5):793–804.
18. Epstein L, Hunter JC, Arwady MA, et al. New Delhi metallo-beta-lactamase-producing carbapenem-resistant Escherichia coli associated with exposure to duodenoscopes. JAMA 2014;312(14):1447–55.
19. Ross AS, Baliga C, Verma P, et al. A quarantine process for the resolution of duodenoscope-associated transmission of multidrug-resistant Escherichia coli. Gastrointest Endosc 2015;82(3):477–83.
20. Smith ZL, Oh YS, Saeian K, et al. Transmission of carbapenem-resistant Enterobacteriaceae during ERCP: time to revisit the current reprocessing guidelines. Gastrointest Endosc 2015;81(4):1041–5.
21. Wendorf KA, Kay M, Baliga C, et al. Endoscopic retrograde cholangiopancreatography-associated AmpC Escherichia coli outbreak. Infect Control Hosp Epidemiol 2015;36(6):634–42.
22. Ray MJ, Lin MY, Tang AS, et al. Regional spread of an outbreak of carbapenem-resistant enterobacteriaceae through an ego network of healthcare facilities. Clin Infect Dis 2018;67(3):407–10.
23. Fraser TG, Reiner S, Malczynski M, et al. Multidrug-resistant Pseudomonas aeruginosa cholangitis after endoscopic retrograde cholangiopancreatography

failure of routine endoscope cultures to prevent an outbreak. Infect Control Hosp Epidemiol 2004;25(10):856–9.

24. Qiu L, Zhou Z, Liu Q, et al. Investigating the failure of repeated standard cleaning and disinfection of a Pseudomonas aeruginosa-infected pancreatic and biliary endoscope. Am J Infect Control 2015;43(8):e43–6.

25. Verfaillie CJ, Bruno MJ, Voor in 't Holt AF, et al. Withdrawal of a novel-design duodenoscope ends outbreak of a VIM-2-producing Pseudomonas aeruginosa. Endoscopy 2015;47(6):493–502.

26. Yetkin FE Y, Kuzucu C, Otlu B, et al. An outbreak associated with multidrug-resistant Pseudomonas aeruginosa contamination of duodenoscopes and an automated endoscope reprocessor. Biomed Res 2017;28(13):6064–70.

27. Robertson P, Smith A, Anderson M, et al. Transmission of Salmonella enteritidis after endoscopic retrograde cholangiopancreatography because of inadequate endoscope decontamination. Am J Infect Control 2017;45(4):440–2.

28. Muscarella LF. Use of ethylene-oxide gas sterilisation to terminate multidrug-resistant bacterial outbreaks linked to duodenoscopes. BMJ Open Gastroenterol 2019;6(1):e000282.

29. Brandabur JJ, Leggett JE, Wang L, et al. Surveillance of guideline practices for duodenoscope and linear echoendoscope reprocessing in a large healthcare system. Gastrointest Endosc 2016;84(3):392–399 e393.

30. Paula H, Presterl E, Tribl B, et al. Microbiologic surveillance of duodenoscope reprocessing at the Vienna University Hospital from November 2004 through March 2015. Infect Control Hosp Epidemiol 2015;36(10):1233–5.

31. Naryzhny I, Silas D, Chi K. Impact of ethylene oxide gas sterilization of duodenoscopes after a carbapenem-resistant Enterobacteriaceae outbreak. Gastrointest Endosc 2016;84(2):259–62.

32. Snyder GM, Wright SB, Smithey A, et al. Randomized Comparison of 3 High-Level Disinfection and Sterilization Procedures for Duodenoscopes. Gastroenterology 2017;153(4):1018–25.

33. Ubhayawardana DL, Kottahachchi J, Weerasekera MM, et al. Residual bioburden in reprocessed side-view endoscopes used for endoscopic retrograde cholangiopancreatography (ERCP). Endosc Int Open 2013;1(1):12–6.

34. U.S. Food and Drug Administration. Duodenoscope surveillance sampling & culturing 2018. Available at: https://www.fda.gov/downloads/MedicalDevices/ProductsandMedicalProcedures/ReprocessingofReusableMedicalDevices/UCM597949.pdf. Accessed March 1, 2018.

35. U.S. Food and Drug Administration. The FDA continues to remind facilities of the importance of following duodenoscope reprocessing instructions: FDA safety communication 2019. Available at: https://www.fda.gov/medical-devices/safety-communications/fda-continues-remind-facilities-importance-following-duodenoscope-reprocessing-instructions-fda. Accessed April 12, 2019.

36. Kramer A, Schwebke I, Kampf G. How long do nosocomial pathogens persist on inanimate surfaces? A systematic review. BMC Infect Dis 2006;6:130.

37. Otter JA, Yezli S, Salkeld JA, et al. Evidence that contaminated surfaces contribute to the transmission of hospital pathogens and an overview of strategies to address contaminated surfaces in hospital settings. Am J Infect Control 2013;41(5 Suppl):S6–11.

38. Paczosa MK, Mecsas J. Klebsiella pneumoniae: going on the offense with a strong defense. Microbiol Mol Biol Rev 2016;80(3):629–61.

39. Piperaki ET, Syrogiannopoulos GA, Tzouvelekis LS, et al. Klebsiella pneumoniae: virulence, biofilm and antimicrobial resistance. Pediatr Infect Dis J 2017;36(10): 1002–5.
40. Kwok K, Chang J, Lo S, et al. A novel adjunctive cleansing method to reduce colony-forming units on duodenoscopes. Endosc Int Open 2016;4(11):E1178–82.
41. Balan GG, Rosca I, Ursu EL, et al. Duodenoscope-associated infections beyond the elevator channel: alternative causes for difficult reprocessing. Molecules 2019;24(12):2343.
42. Pajkos A, Vickery K, Cossart Y. Is biofilm accumulation on endoscope tubing a contributor to the failure of cleaning and decontamination? J Hosp Infect 2004; 58(3):224–9.
43. Kovaleva J. Endoscope drying and its pitfalls. J Hosp Infect 2017;97(4):319–28.
44. Ofstead CL, Heymann OL, Quick MR, et al. Residual moisture and waterborne pathogens inside flexible endoscopes: evidence from a multisite study of endoscope drying effectiveness. Am J Infect Control 2018;46(6):689–96.
45. Humphries RM, McDonnell G. Superbugs on duodenoscopes: the challenge of cleaning and disinfection of reusable devices. J Clin Microbiol 2015;53(10): 3118–25.
46. Kamaruzzaman NF, Tan LP, Mat Yazid KA, et al. Targeting the bacterial protective armour; challenges and novel strategies in the treatment of microbial biofilm. Materials (Basel) 2018;11(9):1705.
47. Adlhart C, Verran J, Azevedo NF, et al. Surface modifications for antimicrobial effects in the healthcare setting: a critical overview. J Hosp Infect 2018;99(3): 239–49.
48. Hawthorn LA, Reid G. Exclusion of uropathogen adhesion to polymer surfaces by Lactobacillus acidophilus. J Biomed Mater Res 1990;24(1):39–46.
49. Lopez AI, Kumar A, Planas MR, et al. Biofunctionalization of silicone polymers using poly(amidoamine) dendrimers and a mannose derivative for prolonged interference against pathogen colonization. Biomaterials 2011;32(19):4336–46.
50. Alfa MJ, Singh H, Nugent Z, et al. Sterile reverse osmosis water combined with friction are optimal for channel and lever cavity sample collection of flexible duodenoscopes. Front Med (Lausanne) 2017;4:191.
51. Cattoir L, Vanzieleghem T, Florin L, et al. Surveillance of endoscopes: comparison of different sampling techniques. Infect Control Hosp Epidemiol 2017;38(9): 1062–9.
52. Gazdik MA, Coombs J, Burke JP, et al. Comparison of two culture methods for use in assessing microbial contamination of duodenoscopes. J Clin Microbiol 2016;54(2):312–6.
53. Archibald LK, Jarvis WR. Health care-associated infection outbreak investigations by the Centers for Disease Control and Prevention, 1946-2005. Am J Epidemiol 2011;174(11 Suppl):S47–64.
54. Sommerstein R, Schreiber PW, Diekema DJ, et al. Mycobacterium chimaera outbreak associated with heater-cooler devices: piecing the puzzle together. Infect Control Hosp Epidemiol 2017;38(1):103–8.
55. Valeriani F, Agodi A, Casini B, et al. Potential testing of reprocessing procedures by real-time polymerase chain reaction: a multicenter study of colonoscopy devices. Am J Infect Control 2018;46(2):159–64.

Antimicrobial Resistance

Lindsay Morrison, MD*, Teresa R. Zembower, MD, MPH

KEYWORDS

- Antimicrobial resistance • Gram-negative resistance • Infection prevention
- Antimicrobial stewardship

KEY POINTS

- Antimicrobial resistance is increasing at an alarming rate.
- Overuse and misuse of antimicrobials leads to increased antimicrobial resistance.
- Preventing the spread of antimicrobial resistance and decreasing antimicrobial use are key factors in slowing the development of antimicrobial resistance.

ANTIMICROBIAL RESISTANCE: BACKGROUND

Given recent media attention, it would be easy to assume that antimicrobial resistance is a new problem; however, antimicrobial resistance has existed well before antimicrobials were identified, synthesized, or commercialized. In fact, bacteria more than 2000 years old isolated from glacial waters carry resistance to ampicillin,[1] and others isolated from permafrost more than 30,000 years old demonstrate resistance to vancomycin.[2] Many of the antibiotics in clinical use today are naturally produced by environmental organisms. Penicillin, for example, is synthesized by a type of mold as a natural defense against bacteria.[3] *Staphylococcus aureus* has been known to have resistance to penicillin antibiotics since the introduction of penicillin into clinical use.[4]

Throughout this article we will discuss anti*microbial* resistance. This term encompasses resistance demonstrated by microbes, which include bacteria, viruses, fungi, and parasites. Anti*biotic* resistance is a term limited to bacteria. Although this article focuses primarily on antibiotic resistance, it is important to note that resistances of all microbes are of clinical and epidemiologic significance.

Worldwide

Globalization has had a significant impact on the spread of antimicrobial resistance.[5] Global trade and travel allow organisms to spread further than ever before. New Delhi Metallo-beta-lactamase 1, an enzyme that confers resistance to a broad array of

Division of Infectious Disease, McGaw Medical Center, Northwestern University Feinberg School of Medicine, 645 North Michigan Avenue, Suite 900, Chicago, IL 60611, USA
* Corresponding author.
E-mail address: lindsay.morrison@northwestern.edu

Gastrointest Endoscopy Clin N Am 30 (2020) 619–635
https://doi.org/10.1016/j.giec.2020.06.004
giendo.theclinics.com

antibiotics, was identified in 2008 in an Indian patient being treated in Sweden.[6] It has now been found on multiple continents with links to travel from or within India.[6] The introduction of foreign antimicrobial resistance provides opportunities for the spread of resistance within local microbial populations. Currently, drug-resistant infections cause at least 700,000 deaths annually. In April 2019, the World Health Organization published a report stating that, if no action is taken, that figure is predicted to increase to 10 million deaths per year by 2050, surpassing diabetes, heart disease, and cancer as the leading cause of death in humans.[7]

United States

Data released in December 2019 demonstrate that in the United States alone, over 2.8 million people acquire drug-resistant infections annually, resulting in over 35,000 deaths with an even larger number of hospitalizations.[8] The economic and human cost of these infections is significant, with estimates that the overall direct costs of healthcare-associated infections (HAIs) to the US healthcare system ranges from 28 to 45 billion dollars per year.[9]

ANTIBIOTIC RESISTANCE: HOW IT DEVELOPS

Owing to the global and increasing threat that antibiotic resistance poses, it is important to first understand the genetic basis of bacterial resistance. For ease of understanding, antibiotic resistance is categorized as either intrinsic or acquired. Intrinsic resistance is a naturally occurring phenomenon that is independent of antibiotic exposure and is universally found within the genome of a group of bacteria or within a bacterial species. This type of resistance is typically chromosomally mediated and can be predicted from an organism's identity.[10] For instance, all *Klebsiella pneumoniae* are intrinsically resistant to ampicillin, all *Enterococcus faecium* and *faecalis* are resistant to cephalosporins, gram-positive cocci are resistant to aztreonam, and gram-negative bacilli are resistant to vancomycin. Traditional mechanisms of intrinsic resistance include lack of outer membrane permeability, which prevents an antibiotic from entering or accumulating inside the bacterial cell; the presence of nonspecific efflux pumps, which expel antibiotics and other substances from inside bacterial cells; or a lack of target sites required by the antibiotic, such that, even if the antibiotic enters the cell, it cannot bind to the target to kill or inhibit the bacteria.[10]

Recent advances in microbial ecology have led the concept of the antibiotic resistome, an environmental reservoir of all antibiotic resistance genes and their precursors in both pathogenic and nonpathogenic bacteria, to explain how intrinsic resistance may develop and spread within bacteria.[11,12] Bacteria that live in soil, most of which are nonpathogenic, are constantly exposed to different chemicals and they have developed mechanisms to interact with other microbes and to defend themselves from threats. Some of the bioactive molecules they produce to protect themselves have led to the evolution of highly specific resistance elements even in the absence of innate antibiotic production. To demonstrate this phenomenon, D'Costa and colleagues[11] isolated a morphologically diverse collection of spore-forming bacteria from soil from diverse locations (urban, agricultural, and forest) and subjected 480 strains to 21 antibiotics that were natural products like vancomycin and erythromycin, semisynthetic derivatives like minocycline and cephalexin, and completely synthetic antibiotics like ciprofloxacin and linezolid. They included older antibiotics and antibiotics that had only been recently introduced to market such as telithromycin and tigecycline. They found that every strain was multidrug-resistant to 7 or 8 antibiotics on average and 2 strains were resistant to 15 antibiotics. They identified almost 200 different resistance profiles. This finding sparked a new field of inquiry into how intrinsic bacterial resistance in environmental reservoirs can lead to resistance in the pathogenic bacteria we see routinely in clinical practice.

Antimicrobial resistance can also be acquired, and this is typically the type of resistance we worry about in clinical practice when we encounter bacteria that were initially susceptible but then become resistant to antibiotics.[13] Many factors play a role in acquired drug resistance, but the main driver is antibiotic overuse. Acquired resistance occurs 1 of 2 ways, either through bacterial gene mutations or through the acquisition of foreign DNA that encodes resistance genes. Bacteria can reproduce rapidly, leading to evolutionary shifts through random genetic mutations that can be seen in relatively short periods of time. Exposure to antibiotics creates an evolutionary pressure on bacteria and confers a selective survival advantage for the bacteria that have acquired the resistance mutations.[14] Alternatively, bacteria can transfer genetic material from 1 cell to another, a process known as horizontal gene transfer.[15] There are 3 traditional processes of horizontal gene transfer: transduction, conjugation, and transformation. Transduction involves genetic material transferred from 1 bacterium to another by a bacterial virus, also known as a bacteriophage. Transformation is the direct uptake of free genetic material from the environment, usually from a lysed bacterial cell. Conjugation, the process most notable for antibiotic resistance, is the process of sharing small segments of DNA directly between cells. Conjugation can involve circular, extra-chromosomal DNA called plasmids, as well as integrative and conjugative elements, which can be integrated into bacterial chromosomes.[15,16] Plasmids can be disseminated rapidly through bacterial communities. These characteristics allow bacteria to not only rapidly develop changes to their genetic material, which may confer resistance, but to also rapidly share this genetic material. Plasmids may also disseminate across bacterial species.[17] For example, the CTX-M beta-lactamase, often linked to resistance in *Escherichia coli*, originated as a plasmid encoded enzyme from environmental *Kluyveyra* strains.[17] In addition to these classic mechanisms of horizontal gene transfer, a variety of other mobile genetic elements exist that can transfer bacterial resistance traits such as genomic islands, insertion sequences, transposons, integrons, and miniature inverted repeat transposable elements.[18]

MECHANISMS OF ANTIBIOTIC RESISTANCE

Apart from knowing the genetic basis of resistance, it is critically important to understand the specific resistance mechanisms if we are to devise effective therapeutic strategies. Generally speaking, there are 4 types of resistance mechanisms. These mechanisms include:

1. Decreased drug accumulation by either decreased outer membrane permeability or increased active efflux of the drugs across the cell surface.
2. Drug inactivation or modification through production of enzymes that either destroy or alter the antibiotic, rendering it ineffective.
3. Alteration of target or binding sites such alteration of penicillin-binding proteins, or alteration of ribosomal-binding proteins.
4. Alteration of metabolic pathways, such as the ability of enterococci to absorb folic acid from the environment, which allows them to bypass the effects of trimethoprim-sulfamethoxazole.

Bacterial species seem to have evolved a preference for 1 type of resistance mechanism over others. For example, penicillin resistance among gram-negative bacteria is predominantly mediated by production of beta-lactamase enzymes that destroy the antibiotic, whereas gram-positive bacteria predominantly modify the penicillin-binding sites to render them penicillin resistant. Specific examples of antibiotic resistance stratified by antibiotic class are reviewed elsewhere in this article and in **Table 1**.

Beta-Lactam Resistance

Beta-lactamases are an important mechanism of resistance in gram-negative bacteria.[19] These enzymes hydrolyze the beta-lactam ring of beta-lactam antibiotics, rendering them ineffective. Beta-lactamases were first described in E coli shortly after the clinical use of penicillin began in the 1940s.[20] These enzymes may be encoded chromosomally or, more often, on plasmids or transposons.[21] The hundreds of beta-lactamases now identified can be organized by their structure, as proposed by Ambler.[22] This classification divides beta-lactamases into 4 groups (A–D). Classes A, C, and D all have serine at their active site, whereas class B, the metallo–beta-lactamases, have zinc at the active site. Beta-lactamases are found primarily in gram-negative bacteria but have also been described in S aureus. Although S aureus possessed beta-lactamase even before the discovery of penicillin, the prevalence of beta-lactamase–producing S aureus increased rapidly after its introduction into clinical use.[23,24]

Beta-lactamase inhibitors such as clavulanic acid, sulbactam, and tazobactam were introduced to overcome the actions of beta-lactamases. These inhibitors work by binding to the active site on the beta-lactamase enzyme, thus preventing binding and hydrolysis of the beta-lactam antibiotic.[25]

Extended spectrum beta-lactamases (ESBLs) confer resistance to a broader array of antibiotics, including, in addition to penicillins, beta-lactams with extended coverage, such as third-generation cephalosporins, and the monobactam aztreonam. Shortly after the introduction of these broad-spectrum antibiotics into clinical practice in the 1980s, the first ESBL was described.[26] Certain beta-lactamases and ESBLs are genetically linked. As an example, the TEM-derived ESBL, the most common ESBL in gram-negative bacteria, differs from the parent TEM beta-lactamase by only 4 amino acids.[27] This small change confers the ability to hydrolyze this broader range of antibiotics.[25,28]

AmpC beta-lactamases have the characteristic of being inducible by the presence of beta-lactam antibiotics. Primarily chromosomally encoded, these enzymes are typically repressed but are transcribed at higher rates in the presence of beta-lactam antibiotics.[29] This type of inducible AmpC beta-lactamase can be seen in several types of bacteria including many Enterobacteriaceae (*Enterobacter* sp., *Citrobacter freundii*, *Serratia* sp., *Providencia* sp., and *Morganella morganii*), *Acinetobacter* sp. and *Pseudomonas aeruginosa*.[29] This induction of AmpC beta-lactamase typically abates once the antibiotic exposure is removed. However, spontaneous mutations may occur, which lead to a "de-repressed state" in which the bacteria continue to produce the beta-lactamase.[30] AmpC beta-lactamases have more recently been described as plasmid-mediated enzymes in several species of bacteria. Genetic analysis has revealed significant similarities to chromosomally encoded AmpC beta-lactamases from *Enterobacteriaceae* or other species, suggesting the chromosomal enzyme was the origin.[31]

Carbapenem Resistance

Carbapenem resistance develops in a number of ways. Carbapenemases, enzymes that can hydrolyze the beta-lactam ring of carbapenems as well as all other beta-lactam antibiotics, are a common mechanism.[32] The most common carbapenemase in the United States is K pneumoniae carbapenemase, an enzyme first identified in K

Table 1
Resistance mechanisms and management

Resistance Class	Most Common Resistance Mechanisms	Drugs to Treat Uncomplicated Infections	Preferred Therapy for Complicated Infections	Detection
Methicillin-resistant *S aureus* (MRSA)	SCCmec contains mecA, which encodes penicillin-binding protein-2a which beta-lactams do not affect	Vancomycin Linezolid Daptomycin Ceftaroline Occasionally: bactrim, minocycline/doxycycline, clindamycin	Vancomycin Linezolid Daptomycin Ceftaroline	mecA genetic testing Routine susceptibility profile and MIC interpretation
Vancomycin-intermediate *S aureus* (VISA)	Adds multiple dipeptides (d-ala-d-ala) to cell wall, thickening cell wall and providing dead end binding sites for vancomycin	Linezolid Ceftaroline Occasionally: minocycline/doxycycline, tigecycline, bactrim, clindamycin	Linezolid Ceftaroline	MRSA isolate with a vancomycin MIC of 4–8 μg/mL
Vancomycin-resistant *S aureus* (VRSA)	Changes end terminal dipeptides from d-ala-d-ala to d-ala-D-serine so vancomycin is unable to bind to the bacteria, mutation via vanA	Linezolid Daptomycin Ceftaroline	Linezolid Daptomycin Ceftaroline	MRSA isolate with a vancomycin MIC of >16 μg/mL
Vancomycin-resistant enterococci (VRE)	Changes end terminal dipeptides from d-ala-d-ala to d-ala-D-serine so vancomycin is unable to bind to the bacteria, mutation via vanA	Linezolid Daptomycin Occasionally: ampicillin, aminoglycosides	Linezolid Daptomycin Occasionally: ampicillin, aminoglycosides	Enterococcus isolate with a vancomycin MIC ≥32 μg/mL

Resistance Class	Resistance Mechanisms	Drugs to Treat Uncomplicated Infections	Preferred Therapy for Complicated Infections	Detection
Extended spectrum beta-lactamases (ESBL) Subtypes: CTX-M, SHV, TEM, OXA	Plasmid-mediated enzyme that hydrolyzes beta-lactam ring of third-generation cephalosporins and monobactams but not carbapenems	Carbapenems Aminoglycosides Fosfomycin Tetracyclines Fluoroquinolones Nitrofurantoin Cefepime Piperacillin-tazobactam Ceftazidime-avibactam Ceftolazone-tazobactam	Carbapenems Ceftazidime-avibactam Ceftolazone-tazobactam Occasionally: fluoroquinolones	Molecular testing Double disk diffusion test using third-generation cephalosporin with and without clavulanic acid
CRE/K pneumoniae carbapenemase Subtypes: Class A (K pneumoniae carbapenemase) Class B (metallo-beta-lactamases) Class C Class D (OXA-type)	Carbapenemases capable of hydrolyzing all beta-lactams including carbapenems	Polymyxins Tigecycline Aztreonam Fosfomycin Nitrofurantoin Aminoglycosides Ceftazidime-avibactam	Combination therapy with or without carbapenem w/: Polymyxins Ceftazidime-avibactam Tigecycline Aztreonam	Molecular testing Modified Hodge test
New Delhi metallo-beta-lactamase	Carbapenemase with zinc at active site, typically more resistant than other classes of carbapenemases	Any susceptible antibiotics Polymyxins Tigecycline	Combination of susceptible antibiotics, occasionally no susceptible antibiotics	Molecular testing
Plasmid-mediated colisitn resistance (MCR-1)	Alteration of cell surface lipid A, leading to poor polymyxin affinity	Any susceptible antibiotics Often with no susceptible antibiotics	Any susceptible antibiotics Often with no susceptible antibiotics	Molecular testing

			Susceptibility testing and MIC interpretation
MDR *Pseudomonas*	Multidrug efflux pumps Change in outer membrane proteins/porins (ie, OprD, a carbapenem specific porin) Change in membrane permeability (resulting in polymyxin resistance) AmpC beta-lactamase Various ESBLs Carbapenemases (most commonly MBLs)	Carbapenems Polymyxins Aminoglycosides Fosfomycin Occasionally: cefepime, piperacillin/tazobactam, fluoroquinolones, aztreonam	CDC/ECDC criteria
MDR *Acinetobacter*	Various carbapenemases (outlined above) AdeABC efflux system Modifications of penicillin-binding proteins Modification of outer membrane proteins (porins)	Aminoglycosides Polymyxins Occasionally: tigecycline. minocycline/doxycycline, ampicillin/sulbactam, fluoroquinolones	Susceptibility testing and MIC interpretation

Abbreviations: CDC, Centers for Disease Control and Prevention; ECDC, European Centre for Disease Prevention and Control; MIC, minimum inhibitory concentration.

pneumoniae, but now found in a number of gram-negative organisms. More recently, additional carbapenemases emerged such as New Delhi metallo-beta-lactamase (NDM), imipenemase metallo-beta-lactamase, and Verona integron-encoded metallo–beta-lactamase. Other mechanisms of carbapenem resistance include the combination of altered membrane permeability and the presence of ESBL enzymes, overexpression of efflux pumps, or, in gram-positive bacteria, alteration of penicillin-binding proteins.[13,32–34]

Trimethoprim-Sulfamethoxazole Resistance

Sulfonamides have been in clinical use as antimicrobial agents since the 1930s with trimethoprim following in the 1960s.[35] Both agents interfere with folic acid synthesis and their combined formulation enhances their activity against a broader array of pathogens.[35]

Quinolone Resistance

Fluoroquinolones are synthetic antibiotics introduced in the 1960s.[36] Several mechanisms of quinolone resistance are known. These include chromosomal mutations causing decreased affinity of the drug targets, DNA gyrase and topoisomerase IV, or overexpression of endogenous efflux pumps.[36] Some organisms can downregulate their porins to decrease bacterial accumulation of drug inside the cell, but this mechanism alone is generally not sufficient to account for high-level fluoroquinolone resistance. Fluoroquinolones quickly developed frequent use after their introduction, aided by their excellent oral bioavailability.[37] Frequent use of fluoroquinolones has led to high worldwide rates of quinolone-resistant microbes.[38]

Aminoglycoside Resistance

Aminoglycosides—antibiotics derived from soil bacteria—bind to the 16s rRNA of the 30s bacterial ribosomal subunit.[39] This disrupts protein production and renders the bacterium dysfunctional. These antibiotics are often considered one of the drugs of last resort in clinical practice owing to their multiple toxicities, including nephrotoxicity and ototoxicity. Resistance to aminoglycosides is primarily conferred by enzymatic modification of the antibiotic as it crosses the bacterial cytoplasmic membrane.[39]

Multidrug Resistance

Bacteria can possess both intrinsic and acquired resistance as well as more than one mechanism of resistance. This can lead to multidrug resistant (MDR), extensively drug resistant, and pan drug resistant bacterial phenotypes. MDR describes bacteria that are resistant to at least 1 antibiotic in 3 or more antibiotic classes, extensively drug resistant describes bacteria that are susceptible to only 1 or 2 antibiotic classes, and pan drug resistant describes bacteria that are not susceptible to any antibiotic class.[40]

Other Types of Antibiotic Resistance

This review is not comprehensive of all antibiotic resistance mechanisms. Other notable types include methicillin-resistant *S aureus*, a frequently encountered pathogen. Methicillin resistance, previously noted mostly in nosocomial *S aureus*, is now frequently encountered in the community.[41] Methicillin-resistant *S aureus* acquires its resistance through an alteration of penicillin-binding proteins.[42] Without the ability to bind to the cell, the antibiotic is ineffective. For each antibiotic available in clinical practice, corresponding resistant bacteria have been described.

esistance Among Other Microbes

Ionbacterial pathogens have shown patterns of resistance to antimicrobials as well. 1 the HIV population, resistant viruses are a well described phenomenon.[43] Fungal organisms may demonstrate resistance to antifungal agents. *Candida glabrata, C krusei,* nd *C lusitanae,* for example, possess intrinsic resistance to certain antifungal agents nd the emerging pathogen, *Candida auris* can be MDR.[44,45]

NTIMICROBIAL RESISTANCE ASSOCIATED WITH GASTROINTESTINAL ENDOSCOPIC ROCEDURES

uodenoscopes represent a potential nidus for the spread of microbes. The human ody is far from a sterile site and plays host to innumerable microbial populations. he gastrointestinal tract in particular is home to a rich community of microbes. Owing) their use within the gastrointestinal tract, duodenoscopes are exposed to many microbes during a single use. These scopes are subsequently cleaned and used again in ther patients. Infection as a result of duodenoscope spread of microbes is uncommon, but does occur on occasion. Recently, there have been reports of the spread f antimicrobial-resistant bacterial populations between patients via duodenoscopy.

nterobacteriaceae

1 2013, a hospital in Illinois identified a highly drug resistant New Delhi metallo-beta-actamase–producing *E coli* in a patient with no history of foreign travel with ubsequent identification of 8 additional colonized patients.[46] Endoscopic retrograde holangiopancreatography was identified as a significant risk factor. Subsequent creening of patients exposed to the duodenoscopes that were identified in the initial luster revealed an additional 30 patients with the New Delhi metallo-beta-lactamase arbapenemase.

seudomonas

aeruginosa is a commonly identified pathogen in hospital settings and is a major ause of health care-associated infections, including endoscopic procedure related fection.[47,48] It is also commonly isolated in non-health care environments such as ot tubs, pools, soil, and vegetation.[48,49] *P aeruginosa* is clinically challenging to treat ecause it possesses intrinsic antibiotic resistance as well as acquired resistance.[50] *seudomonas* sp. often carry multiple types of resistance mechanisms and MDR, xtensively drug-resistant, and pan drug-resistant *Pseudomonas* sp. have been escribed.

almonella

almonella sp. causes a variety of infections in humans but may also cause asymp- omatic carriage within the gastrointestinal tract. *Salmonella* sp. infections transmitted ia endoscopy have been reported and multiple serotypes have been identified.[51]

ther Pathogens

lthough the gram-negative bacteria listed elsewhere in this article have caused the najority of outbreaks after endoscopic procedures, other pathogens have been impli- ated infrequently. The bacteria, *Helicobacter pylori* and *Methylobacterium mesophi- cum*; viruses including both hepatitis B and hepatitis C; the fungi, *Trichosporon* sahii; and the parasite, *Strongyloides stercoralis*, have all been cited as causing single fections or outbreaks after gastrointestinal endoscopy.[51–53]

MANAGING ANTIMICROBIAL RESISTANCE

Antibiotic use drives the evolution of resistance. It has been apparent since the intro duction of antibiotics into clinical practice that development of new antibiotics car never keep pace with the emergence of resistance. Each antibiotic introduction is fol lowed, relatively quickly, by documented resistance to that antibiotic (**Fig. 1**).[54] Thus the primary way to decrease antibiotic resistance is to promote judicious antibiotic use. One arena where this is critically important is in the health care setting, where heavy consumers of antimicrobials, many of whom are immunocompromised, are ir close proximity, providing ongoing selective pressure for the development of resis tance and the milieu for organism transmission and outbreaks. However, we canno lose sight of other important arenas that use antimicrobials in large quantities, suct as the agricultural industry. Notably, the use of antimicrobials in agriculture not only provides evolutionary pressures to drive the development of resistance, but also pro vides a link in the chain of the transmission of resistance genes via spread to ground water, as well as through human ingestion.[55]

Combination Therapy and Drugs of Last Resort

Despite the development of antimicrobial resistance, several existing antibiotics retair their clinical usefulness against MDR bacteria. Many of these are very broad-spectrun antibiotics or antibiotics that had fallen out of routine use owing to their adverse effec profiles. Together these drugs are referred to as drugs of last resort. For example, a resistant bacterium may retain susceptibility to aminoglycosides, notorious for thei nephrotoxic and ototoxic effects. **Table 2** describes common drugs of last resor and their adverse effect profiles.

Combinations of antibiotics may also be clinically useful in the management of anti microbial resistant infections. In vitro and animal model studies have shown promising results with combination therapy for antibiotic resistant bacteria.[56–58] One multicente study in Italy found a lower 30-day mortality in patients with *Klebsiella pneumoniae* carbapenemase–producing *K pneumonia* bloodstream infections who received com bination therapy of 2 or more antibiotics in comparison with those who received mono therapy.[59] A more recent multicenter randomized, controlled trial did not identify a benefit of colistin plus meropenem over colistin alone for patients with carbapenem resistant *Acinetobater baumanii* infections. More studies are needed to determine the safety and efficacy of combination therapy in the treatment of antimicrobial resis tant infections.[60]

Antimicrobial Stewardship Programs

Antimicrobial Stewardship Programs (ASPs) have been implemented in health care settings to help combat antimicrobial resistance. These programs monitor and guide the use of antimicrobials within an institution. In 2015, both the Centers for Medicare and Medicaid Services and the Joint Commission developed standards for ASPs fo health care settings that were put into effect in 2017.[61] The role of ASPs is outlined ir **Box 1**. ASPs develop protocols and guidelines for appropriate antibiotic use. These are drafted with the hospital's unique bacterial populations in mind. The ASPs also participate in clinician and medical staff education on appropriate antibiotic use Importantly, ASPs also play a role in restricting the use of antibiotics. These vary by institution but may include necessitating approval by ASP personnel or obtaining consultation with an infectious disease specialist to use broad spectrum antibi otics.[62] Antimicrobial stewardship teams may also help track the patterns of micro bial resistance seen within the institution by creating an antibiogram of the

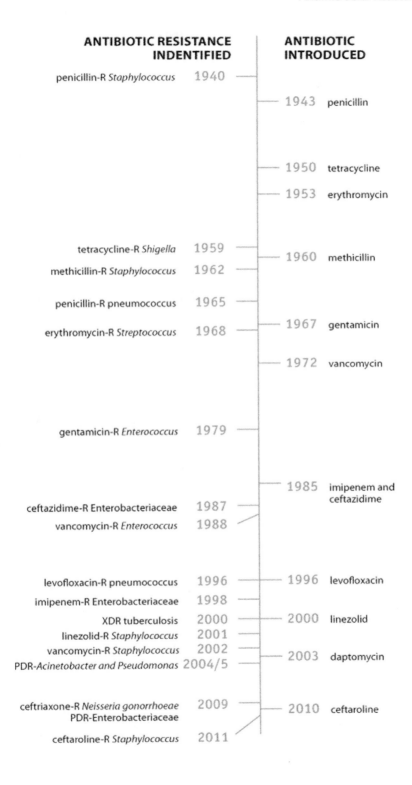

ANTIBIOTIC RESISTANCE INDENTIFIED

ANTIBIOTIC INTRODUCED

penicillin-R *Staphylococcus* 1940

1943 penicillin

1950 tetracycline

1953 erythromycin

tetracycline-R *Shigella* 1959

1960 methicillin

methicillin-R *Staphylococcus* 1962

penicillin-R pneumococcus 1965

1967 gentamicin

erythromycin-R *Streptococcus* 1968

1972 vancomycin

gentamicin-R *Enterococcus* 1979

1985 imipenem and ceftazidime

ceftazidime-R Enterobacteriaceae 1987

vancomycin-R *Enterococcus* 1988

levofloxacin-R pneumococcus 1996

1996 levofloxacin

imipenem-R Enterobacteriaceae 1998

XDR tuberculosis 2000

2000 linezolid

linezolid-R *Staphylococcus* 2001

vancomycin-R *Staphylococcus* 2002

2003 daptomycin

PDR-*Acinetobacter and Pseudomonas* 2004/5

ceftriaxone-R *Neisseria gonorrhoeae* 2009

PDR-Enterobacteriaceae

2010 ceftaroline

ceftaroline-R *Staphylococcus* 2011

institution. This antibiogram is essential for the ASP to draft its guidelines and develop its antibiotic use restrictions. For example, if a health care institution has high rates of fluoroquinolone resistance in its *P aeruginosa* isolates, it may choose not to restrict antipseudomonal cephalosporins because these agents may be a better initial therapeutic choice.

Infection Control and Prevention

In addition to ASPs, health care institutions employ epidemiology teams to monitor for and quickly address outbreaks within an institution. An epidemiologist may routinely monitor the rates of certain types of infections or environmental isolates. When an infection rate deviates from the norm or when a pathogen known to cause outbreaks is identified, the epidemiologist plays a central role in identifying the source and implementing measures to limit further spread. Let us use the example of a *P aeruginosa* outbreak after endoscopic retrograde cholangiopancreatography. The infection prevention personnel would first verify that an outbreak actually exists. If so, they would collect case data to identify patients involved, would implement control measures to limit further infection transmission, and would investigate potential causes, such as the use of contaminated solutions, inadequate instrument cleaning, reprocessing and sterilization, and inadequate rinsing, drying, and storage of instruments. They may then implement surveillance procedures, such as ongoing scope cultures or prospective electronic monitoring for bacteremia for all patients who have recently undergone endoscopy. They would work closely with endoscopy personnel throughout and after the outbreak to control this and to prevent future recurrences.

Novel Antimicrobials

The development of new antimicrobial therapies is essential for treatment of resistant microbes. As illustrated elsewhere in this article, the use of antibiotics serves as a selective pressure for the development of resistance. As new therapies are introduced, new resistance emerges, and new therapies are needed. Novel antimicrobials offer some potential to circumvent existing resistance mechanisms. Most often, these are created by modification of existing antibiotics. Recently, this method has been applied to certain beta-lactams. For example, meropenem/vaborbactam combines a novel beta-lactamase inhibitor with an existing carbapenem antibiotic, and ceftolozane/tazobactam combines a novel cephalosporin with an existing beta-lactamase inhibitor.[63,64] Pharmaceutical developers face regulatory challenges when developing new antimicrobial agents.[65] They are also faced with the paradoxic reality that newly introduced antimicrobials will be used as little as possible to avoid creating selective pressure for resistance. To ensure an antimicrobial gets to market quickly enough to be financially viable, many new therapies rely on modification of existing therapies.[65]

Alternative Therapies

Alternatives to antimicrobials may offer the potential to alleviate the selective pressure of antimicrobial therapy. In the setting of growing antimicrobial resistance, phage

Fig. 1. Timeline of antibiotic introduction compared to early literature documenting antibiotic resistance. (*From* CDC. What exactly is antibiotic resistance? Centers for Disease Control and Prevention. https://www.cdc.gov/drugresistance/about.html. Published March 20, 2019. Accessed September 26, 2019.)

Table 2
Common adverse drug reactions of antimicrobials used to treat resistant infections

Class of Drug	Antimicrobials	Most Common Adverse Events
Aminoglycosides	Amikacin, gentamicin, tobramycin	Renal toxicity (10%–20%), ototoxicity (vestibular and cochlear)
Beta-lactam/ beta-lactamase inhibitors	Ceftazidime-avibactam Ceftolazone-tazobactam	Anxiety, dizziness, constipation Headache, nausea
Carbapenems	Doripenem, imipenem, meropenem, ertapenem[a]	Lowers seizure threshold
Fluoroquinolones	Ciprofloxacin, levofloxacin	QT interval prolongation, tendon rupture with prolonged use
Glycopeptides	Vancomycin	Red man syndrome, dose-dependent nephrotoxicity, reversible neutropenia
Glycylcyclines	Tigecycline	Nausea, vomiting, diarrhea
Lipopeptides	Daptomycin	Increased creatinine phosphokinase, myopathy
Oxazolidinones	Linezolid	Thrombocytopenia, optic neuritis with prolonged use, serotonin syndrome
Polymyxins	Colistin (polymyxin E), polymyxin B	Nephrotoxicity ($\geq$40%), neurotoxicity (confusion, vertigo, parasthesias)
Streptogramins	Quinupristin-dalfopristin	Pain/edema at infusion site ($\geq$45%), arthralgias/myalgias ($\geq$50%), hyperbilirubinemia ($\geq$35%)
Tetracyclines	Doxycycline, minocycline	Phototoxicity, abdominal pain, nausea, vomiting
Other	Fosfomycin, nitrofurantoin	Diarrhea, headache Pulmonary fibrosis with prolonged use

Ertapenem's spectrum of activity differs from other carbapenems. It is ineffective against Enterococcus, Acinetobacter, and Pseudomonas spp.

Box 1
ASPs

- Track antimicrobial prescribing and resistance patterns
- Reporting resistance and prescribing information back to health care teams
  - Example: publicly available institutional antibiogram
- Educating health care teams about resistance and prescribing best practice
  - Example: institutional guidelines for antimicrobial use based on indication and institutional antibiogram
- Implement policies that support optimal antimicrobial use
  - Example: approval of experts required to use broad spectrum antimicrobials
  - Example: checklist completion before prescribing an antimicrobial
- Implement interventions to improve antimicrobial use
  - Example: pharmacist-driven dose adjustment based on patient-specific parameters
  - Example: suggested change from intravenous to oral antibiotic where appropriate

Form Core Elements of Hospital Antibiotic Stewardship Programs | Antibiotic Use | CDC. 5 Aug. 2019, https://www.cdc.gov/antibiotic-use/core-elements/hospital.html.

therapy has garnered renewed interest. Bacteriophages are viruses that selectivel infect bacterial cells. Phage therapy has been investigated as early as th 1920s.[66,67] More recent studies from Eastern Europe have demonstrated efficacy phage therapy in treating several types of drug-resistant gram-negative infection but more rigorous research is still needed.[67] Additional therapies under investigatio include vaccination, immune stimulation, topical agents, and probiotics.[68]

SUMMARY

Antimicrobial resistance poses a major threat to our patients, health care systems an global economy. Bacteria develop antibiotic resistance through a variety of mecha nisms and multidrug resistance among bacteria is now the rule rather than the excep tion. Widespread antibiotic use is the key driver of emerging resistance. Combatin the spread will require multidisciplinary efforts to limit unnecessary antibiotic us and to implement prevention and control measures to limit transmission of thes dangerous pathogens.

DISCLOSURE

The authors have nothing to disclose.

REFERENCES

1. Dancer SJ, Shears P, Platt DJ. Isolation and characterization of coliforms fror glacial ice and water in Canada's High Arctic. J Appl Microbiol 1997;82(5 597–609.
2. D'Costa VM, King CE, Kalan L, et al. Antibiotic resistance is ancient. Nature 201 477(7365):457–61.
3. Ligon BL. Penicillin: its discovery and early development. Semin Pediatr Infec Dis 2004;15(1):52–7.
4. Spink WW, Ferris V. Penicillin-resistant staphylococci: mechanisms involved in th development of resistance. J Clin Invest 1947;26(3):379–93.
5. MacPherson DW. Population mobility, globalization, and antimicrobial drug resis tance. Emerg Infect Dis 2009. https://doi.org/10.3201/eid1511.090419.
6. Nordmann P, Naas T, Poirel L. Global Spread of carbapenemase-producin, Enterobacteriaceae. Emerg Infect Dis 2011;17(10):1791–8.
7. Interagency Coordination Group on Antimicrobial Resistance. No time to wai securing the future from drug-resistant infections. Report to the Secretar General of the United Nations. 2019. Available at: https://www.who.in antimicrobial-resistance/interagency-coordination-group/final-report/en/.   Ac cessed October 10, 2019.
8. CDC. Antibiotic Resistance Threats in the United States, 2019. Atlanta (GA): U.S Department of Health and Human Services, CDC; 2019. p. 3, 89, 97.
9. Stone PW. Economic burden of healthcare-associated infections: an America perspective. Expert Rev Pharmacoecon Outcomes Res 2009;9(5):417–22.
10. Cox G, Wright GD. Intrinsic antibiotic resistance: mechanisms, origins, chal lenges and solutions. Int J Med Microbiol 2013;303(6-7):287–92.
11. D'Costa VM, McGrann KM, Hughes DW, et al. Sampling the antibiotic resistome Science 2006;311(5759):374–7.
12. Gaze WH, Krone SM, Larsson DGJ, et al. Influence of humans on evolution an mobilization of environmental antibiotic resistome. Emerg Infect Dis 2013;19(7 https://doi.org/10.3201/eid1907.120871.

13. Munita JM, Arias CA. Mechanisms of antibiotic resistance. In: Kudva IT, Cornick NA, Plummer PJ, et al, editors. Virulence mechanisms of bacterial pathogens. 5th edition. Sterling (VA): American Society of Microbiology; 2016. p. 481–511.

14. Oz T, Guvenek A, Yildiz S, et al. Strength of selection pressure is an important parameter contributing to the complexity of antibiotic resistance evolution. Mol Biol Evol 2014;31(9):2387–401.

15. Gillings MR, Paulsen IT, Tetu SG. Genomics and the evolution of antibiotic resistance: genomics and antibiotic resistance. Ann N Y Acad Sci 2017;1388(1): 92–107.

16. Oliveira PH, Touchon M, Cury J, et al. The chromosomal organization of horizontal gene transfer in bacteria. Nat Commun 2017;8(1):841.

17. Davies J, Davies D. Origins and evolution of antibiotic resistance. Microbiol Mol Biol Rev 2010;74(3):417–33.

18. Domingues S, da Silva GJ, Nielsen KM. Integrons: vehicles and pathways for horizontal dissemination in bacteria. Mob Genet Elements 2012;2(5):211–23.

19. Wilke MS, Lovering AL, Strynadka NC. β-Lactam antibiotic resistance: a current structural perspective. Curr Opin Microbiol 2005;8(5):525–33.

20. Abraham EP, Chain E. An enzyme from bacteria able to destroy penicillin. Rev Infect Dis 1988;10(4):677–8.

21. Dever LA. Mechanisms of bacterial resistance to antibiotics. Arch Intern Med 1991;151(5):886.

22. Ambler RP. The structure of beta-lactamases. Philos Trans R Soc Lond B Biol Sci 1980;289(1036):321–31.

23. Livermore DM. Beta-lactamases in laboratory and clinical resistance. Clin Microbiol Rev 1995;8(4):557–84.

24. Bradford PA. Extended-spectrum -lactamases in the 21st century: characterization, epidemiology, and detection of this important resistance threat. Clin Microbiol Rev 2001;14(4):933–51.

25. Babic M, Hujer A, Bonomo R. What's new in antibiotic resistance? Focus on beta-lactamases. Drug Resist Updat 2006;9(3):142–56.

26. Kliebe C, Nies BA, Meyer JF, et al. Evolution of plasmid-coded resistance to broad-spectrum cephalosporins. Antimicrob Agents Chemother 1985;28(2): 302–7.

27. Sougakoff W, Petit A, Goussard S, et al. Characterization of the plasmid genes blaT-4 and blaT-5 which encode the broad-spectrum β-lactamases TEM-4 and TEM-5 in Enterobacteriaceae. Gene 1989;78(2):339–48.

28. Philippon A, Labia R, Jacoby G. Extended-spectrum beta-lactamases. Antimicrob Agents Chemother 1989;33(8):1131–6.

29. Jones RN. Important and emerging β-lactamase-mediated resistances in hospital-based pathogens: the amp c enzymes. Diagn Microbiol Infect Dis 1998;31(3):461–6.

30. Sanders CC. Novel resistance selected by the new expanded-spectrum cephalosporins: a concern. J Infect Dis 1983;147(3):585–9.

31. Philippon A, Arlet G, Jacoby GA. Plasmid-determined AmpC-type -lactamases. Antimicrob Agents Chemother 2002;46(1):1–11.

32. Potter RF, D'Souza AW, Dantas G. The rapid spread of carbapenem-resistant Enterobacteriaceae. Drug Resist Updat 2016;29:30–46.

33. Li X-Z, Plésiat P, Nikaido H. The challenge of efflux-mediated antibiotic resistance in gram-negative bacteria. Clin Microbiol Rev 2015;28(2):337–418.

34. Livermore DM. Interplay of impermeability and chromosomal beta-lactamase activity in imipenem-resistant *Pseudomonas aeruginosa*. Antimicrob Agents Chemother 1992;36(9):2046–8.
35. Eliopoulos GM, Huovinen P. Resistance to trimethoprim-sulfamethoxazole. Clin Infect Dis 2001;32(11):1608–14.
36. Ruiz J, Pons MJ, Gomes C. Transferable mechanisms of quinolone resistance. Int J Antimicrob Agents 2012;40(3):196–203.
37. Davis R, Markham A, Balfour JA. Ciprofloxacin: an updated review of its pharmacology, therapeutic efficacy and tolerability. Drugs 1996;51(6):1019–74.
38. Acar JF, Goldstein FW. Trends in bacterial resistance to fluoroquinolones. Clin Infect Dis 1997;24(Supplement_1):S67–73.
39. Doi Y, Wachino J, Arakawa Y. Aminoglycoside resistance. Infect Dis Clin North Am 2016;30(2):523–37.
40. Magiorakos A-P, Srinivasan A, Carey RB, et al. Multidrug-resistant, extensively drug-resistant and pandrug-resistant bacteria: an international expert proposal for interim standard definitions for acquired resistance. Clin Microbiol Infect 2012;18(3):268–81.
41. Ray SM. Preventing methicillin-resistant staphylococcus aureus (MRSA) disease in urban US hospitals – now for the hard part: more evidence pointing to the community as the source of MRSA acquisition. J Infect Dis 2017;215(11):1631–3.
42. Hassoun A, Linden PK, Friedma B. Incidence, prevalence, and management of MRSA bacteremia across patient populations-a review of recent developments in MRSA management and treatment. Crit Care 2017;21(1):211.
43. Wainberg MA. Public health implications of antiretroviral therapy and HIV drug resistance. JAMA 1998;279(24):1977.
44. Perlin DS, Rautemaa-Richardson R, Alastruey-Izquierdo A. The global problem of antifungal resistance: prevalence, mechanisms, and management. Lancet Infect Dis 2017;17(12):e383–92.
45. Chowdhary A, Voss A, Meis JF. Multidrug-resistant Candida auris: "new kid on the block" in hospital-associated infections? J Hosp Infect 2016;94(3):209–12.
46. Epstein L, Hunter JC, Arwady MA, et al. New Delhi metallo-β-lactamase–producing carbapenem-resistant *Escherichia coli* associated with exposure to duodenoscopes. JAMA 2014;312(14):1447.
47. Doherty DE, Falko JM, Lefkovitz N, et al. Pseudomonas aeruginosa sepsis following retrograde cholangiopancreatography (ERCP). Dig Dis Sci 1982; 27(2):169–70.
48. Lister PD, Wolter DJ, Hanson ND. Antibacterial-resistant pseudomonas aeruginosa: clinical impact and complex regulation of chromosomally encoded resistance mechanisms. Clin Microbiol Rev 2009;22(4):582–610.
49. Green SK, Schroth MN, Cho JJ, et al. Agricultural plants and soil as a reservoir for Pseudomonas aeruginosa. Appl Microbiol 1974;28(6):987–91.
50. Bonomo RA, Szabo D. Mechanisms of multidrug resistance in Acinetobacter species and pseudomonas aeruginosa. Clin Infect Dis 2006;43(Supplement_2): S49–56.
51. Spach DH. Transmission of infection by gastrointestinal endoscopy and bronchoscopy. Ann Intern Med 1993;118(2):117.
52. Calderwood AH, Day LW, Muthusamy VR, et al. ASGE guideline for infection control during GI endoscopy. Gastrointest Endosc 2018;87(5):1167–79.
53. Kovaleva J, Peters FTM, van der Mei HC, et al. Transmission of infection by flexible gastrointestinal endoscopy and bronchoscopy. Clin Microbiol Rev 2013; 26(2):231–54.

4. CDC. What exactly is antibiotic resistance? Centers for Disease Control and Prevention. 2019. Available at: https://www.cdc.gov/drugresistance/about.html. Accessed September 26, 2019.

5. Manyi-Loh C, Mamphweli S, Meyer E, et al. Antibiotic use in agriculture and its consequential resistance in environmental sources: potential public health implications. Molecules 2018;23(4). https://doi.org/10.3390/molecules23040795.

6. Paul M, Daikos GL, Durante-Mangoni E, et al. Colistin alone versus colistin plus meropenem for treatment of severe infections caused by carbapenem-resistant Gram-negative bacteria: an open-label, randomised controlled trial. Lancet Infect Dis 2018;18(4):391–400.

7. Nath S, Moussavi F, Abraham D, et al. In vitro and in vivo activity of single and dual antimicrobial agents against KPC-producing *Klebsiella pneumoniae*. J Antimicrob Chemother 2018;73(2):431–6.

8. Bulik CC, Nicolau DP. Double-carbapenem therapy for carbapenemase-producing *Klebsiella pneumoniae*. Antimicrob Agents Chemother 2011;55(6): 3002–4.

9. Yim J, Smith JR, Rybak MJ. Role of combination antimicrobial therapy for vancomycin-resistant *Enterococcus faecium* infections: review of the current evidence. Pharmacotherapy 2017;37(5):579–92.

10. Tumbarello M, Viale P, Viscoli C, et al. Predictors of mortality in bloodstream infections caused by Klebsiella pneumoniae carbapenemase-producing K. pneumoniae: importance of combination therapy. Clin Infect Dis 2012;55(7):943–50.

11. Joint Commission Perspectives®, July 2016, Volume 36, Issue 7 Copyright 2016 The Joint Commission. Available at: https://www.jointcommission.org/new_antimicrobial_stewardship_standard/. Accessed September 12, 2019.

12. Core elements of hospital antibiotic stewardship programs. Antibiotic Use. CDC. 2019. Available at: https://www.cdc.gov/antibiotic-use/core-elements/hospital.html. Accessed September 9, 2019.

13. Cho JC, Zmarlicka MT, Shaeer KM, et al. Meropenem/vaborbactam, the first carbapenem/beta-lactamase inhibitor combination. Ann Pharmacother 2018; 52(8):769–79.

14. Van Duin D, Bonomo RA. Ceftazidime/avibactam and ceftolozane/tazobactam: second-generation beta-lactam/beta-lactamase inhibitor combinations. Clin Infect Dis 2016;63(2):234–41.

15. Simpkin VL, Renwick MJ, Kelly R, et al. Incentivising innovation in antibiotic drug discovery and development: progress, challenges and next steps. J Antibiot 2017;70(12):1087–96.

16. Kutter E, Sulakvelidze A, editors. Bacteriophages: biology and applications. Boca Raton (FL): CRC Press; 2005.

17. Sulakvelidze A, Alavidze Z, Morris JG. Bacteriophage therapy. Antimicrob Agents Chemother 2001;45(3):649–59.

18. Renwick MJ, Simpkin V, Mossialos E. World Health Organization, Regional Office for Europe, European Observatory on Health systems and policies. Targeting Innovation in antibiotic drug discovery and development: the need for a one Health - one Europe - one World Framework 2016. Available at: http://www.ncbi.nlm.nih.gov/books/NBK447337/. Accessed October 11, 2019.

Nosocomial Infections
A History of Hospital-Acquired Infections

Jia-Yia Liu, MD[a,b,c],*, Jana K. Dickter, MD[d]

KEYWORDS

- Health care acquired • Nosocomial • Pneumonia • Urinary tract • Bloodstream
- Surgical site

KEY POINTS

- Sixth leading cause of death in the United States.
- 99,000 annual deaths.
- Contributes to multidrug-resistant organisms.
- Most infections are preventable.

INTRODUCTION

In the United States, health-care acquired infections (HAIs) or nosocomial infections (NIs) are the sixth leading cause of death, surpassing the combined deaths from human immunodeficiency virus/AIDS, cancer, and traffic accidents.[1,2] Since Hippocrates's time, physicians have been aware HAIs harm patients.[1] HAIs refer to infections that arise in any inpatient or outpatient setting and appear 48 hours after hospitalization, or within 30 days after receiving health care, or up to 90 days after undergoing certain surgical procedures.[1,3,4] The highest at-risk population are patients who are immunocompromised, such as transplant patients, chemotherapy patients, and neonates, and critically ill admitted to burn units or intensive care units (ICUs).[5] In 2002, there were 1.7 million NIs, approximately 99,000 hospitalized patients who died of NIs, and 1 in 31 hospitalized patients per day developed an NI.[2,6,7] The direct economic burden of HAIs in the United States is estimated to be between $28 and $34 billion, of which $25 to $32 billion could be prevented with effective infection-control programs.[8]

To combat and reduce HAIs, the Centers for Disease Control and Prevention (CDC) National Healthcare Safety Network (NHSN) and the Centers for Medicare and

[a] American Medical Physicians and Surgeons Advancement Alliance; [b] Department of Medicine, Loma Linda University, Loma Linda, CA, USA; [c] Division of Infectious Diseases, Cedars-Sinai Medical Center, Los Angeles, CA, USA; [d] Division of Infectious Diseases, City of Hope, 1500 East Duarte Road, Duarte, CA 91010, USA
* Corresponding author. 19069 Van Buren Boulevard, Ste 114-406, Riverside, CA 92508.
E-mail address: Jia-Yia.Liux@cshs.org

Gastrointest Endoscopy Clin N Am 30 (2020) 637–652
https://doi.org/10.1016/j.giec.2020.06.001
1052-5157/20/© 2020 Elsevier Inc. All rights reserved.

Medicaid Services implemented programs to monitor and reduce the rates of NIs.[9] The NHSN is now the largest tracking system of HAIs in the United States and includes 25,000 medical facilities spanning across 50 states and US territories.[10,11] This is an improvement compared with the mid-1970s, when only 62 US hospitals participated in programs to reduce HAIs.[11,12]

Catheter-associated urinary tract infections (CAUTIs), hospital-acquired pneumonias (HAPs), bloodstream infections (BSIs), and surgical site infections (SSIs) cause most HAIs.[5] Among them, CAUTIs are the most prevalent worldwide NIs, causing 40% of all US NIs or 900,000 cases annually.[5,13] However, the most deadly NIs are HAPs and BSIs, which together account for 67% of US annual deaths associated with NIs.[14] Lower tract urinary infections are often the precursor for upper tract urinary infections and BSIs. Urinary tract infections are the leading cause of secondary bacteremia and account for 17% of nosocomial bacteremias.[13,15]

A significant factor in the rising mortality of NIs is the increasing prevalence of multidrug-resistant organisms (MDROs), which can render classes of antibiotics ineffective in treating many common infectious diseases. Annually more than 2 million people acquire an antibiotic-resistant infection, and of those, 23,000 die.[12,16] These organisms can survive on inanimate surfaces for prolonged periods, contaminate hospital rooms and equipment, and are spread by the hands of health care workers.[17–20] ICU patients are disproportionately affected because of chronic comorbid diseases, more aggressive interventional treatments with indwelling devices, and frequent exposure to antibiotics. The mortality rate of ICU patients is estimated to be more than twice that of non-ICU patients.[21] Aerobic gram-negative bacteria (GNB) account for 40% of all ICU deaths and 70% of all ICU HAIs.[22] GNB have become the most drug resistant because of lack of development of new antimicrobials. The last novel class of antibiotics against GNB was released in 1996: the fluoroquinolones. Several risk factors are associated with acquiring MDROs including prior antibiotic use, septic shock, and 5 or more days of hospitalization.[23]

In this article we focus on the history, prevalence, economic costs, morbidity and mortality, along with risk factors of the most common HAIs; address the emergence of MDROs, including *Staphylococcus aureus* (SA) and *Clostridium difficile*; and discuss examples of effective programs that can reduce infection risks.

NOSOCOMIAL URINARY TRACT INFECTIONS

Nosocomial urinary tract infections are the most common HAIs reported to the NHSN, European Center for Disease Prevention and Control, and the World Health Organization.[24] Most nosocomial urinary tract infections are caused by instrumentation of the urinary tract with either urethral or suprapubic catheters.[13,24] CAUTIs account for 75% of HAIs.[13] Between 15% and 25% of hospitalized patients have indwelling urinary catheters inserted during their hospitalization[13] and many are often inappropriately placed.[25] The highest risk factor for developing CAUTIs is prolonged catheter use.[13,26] Catheter colonization increases the risk of bacteriuria by 3% to 10% per day.[13] After 30 days, 100% of catheters become colonized with a biofilm, where organisms exist in a protected state from antimicrobials and host defenses. The only effective eradication is removal of the catheter.[24,27]

Diagnosis of CAUTIs requires the presence of an indwelling or suprapubic catheter plus infectious signs or symptoms and a positive urine culture. Among patients who develop bacteriuria only 10% to 25% are symptomatic.[24,28] Asymptomatic bacteriuria in catheterized patients, even in the presence of malodorous, cloudy urine and bacteria growth, do not have CAUTI and do not require antimicrobial therapy.[26]

Over the past few years, NHSN reported declining use of urinary catheters, which as reduced CAUTI rate. Prevention strategies included decreasing unnecessary atheter placement, limiting the duration of catheterization, securing closed drainage ystems, and encouraging aseptic technique with only trained personnel performing atheter insertion. **Figs. 1** and **2** demonstrate improvement over the past several years n CAUTI rates.[9]

EALTH CARE–ASSOCIATED PNEUMONIAS

lealth care–associated pneumonias (HCAPs) are the second most common HAI; owever, it is the most deadly.[22,23,29] Every 5 to 10 hospitalized patients out of 000 develop HCAP. Patients with the highest risks of acquiring HCAPs include in-ints; young children; adults older than 65 years of age; and patients who are venti-ited, immunosuppressed, have decreased sensorium, recent thoracoabdominal urgery, and cardiopulmonary disease.[29] HCAPs, which cause 86% of NIs, are ivided into HAPs, which occur after 48 hours of admission, and ventilator-acquired neumonias.[14] The latter causes 86% of all HCAPs.[5] Between 9% and 27% of me-hanically assisted patients are at risk for ventilator-acquired pneumonia within 8 hours after endotracheal intubation.[1,5] HCAP account for 22% of all ICU NIs and re directly associated with prolonged hospitalizations, rising costs, and increased nortality and morbidity.[1,14,23,30] MDROs frequently cause ventilator-acquired pneu-nonia, which is also a major factor in morbidity and mortality.[23] There are several nethods to prevent HCAP, including pneumococcal vaccination, use of incentive pirometry, and chest physiotherapy.[29]

The diagnosis for HCAPs is challenging in patients with comorbid conditions and re-uires documentation of multiple nonspecific clinical factors including fever, cough, roductive sputum, and radiologic evidence of an infiltrate.[23] HCAP pathogens are ften the intrinsic colonizing oral flora of patients. The natural human oral flora is

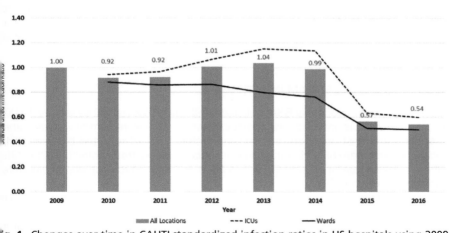

ig. 1. Changes over time in CAUTI standardized infection ratios in US hospitals using 2009 aseline, NHSN 2009 to 2016. SIR, standardized infection ratios. (*Data from*: Centers for Dis-ase Control and Prevention. Data Summary of HAIs in the US: Assessing Progress 2006-2016. ttps://www.cdc.gov/hai/data/archive/data-summary-assessing-progress.html?CDC_AA_ ɛfVal=https%3A%2F%2Fwww.cdc.gov%2Fhai%2Fsurveillance%2Fdata-reports%2Fdata-ʋmmary-assessing-progress.html. Updated December 5, 2017. Accessed September 18, 019.)

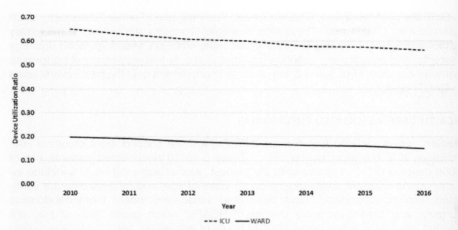

Fig. 2. Changes over time catheter use ratio in US hospitals, 2010 to 2016. (*Data from*: Centers for Disease Control and Prevention. Data Summary of HAIs in the US: Assessing Progress 2006-2016. https://www.cdc.gov/hai/data/archive/data-summary-assessing-progress.html? CDC_AA_refVal=https%3A%2F%2Fwww.cdc.gov%2Fhai%2Fsurveillance%2Fdata-reports %2Fdata-summary-assessing-progress.html. Updated December 5, 2017. Accessed September 18, 2019.)

composed of a healthy mixed population of gram-positive, gram-negative, and anaerobic bacteria, which changes because of several factors including age, chronic illness, orthodontic procedures, antibiotic exposure, and hospitalization.[23,31] Aerobic GNB account for greater than 73% of HCAP cases and frequently respiratory samples are polymicrobial.[23,29]

Interventions minimizing HCAPs include preventing aspiration, sterilization of respiratory devices, aggressive hand hygiene, and reducing GNB colonization through oral care.[19] In 2017, NHSN showed a 5% statistically significant decrease in ventilator-associated events, which was an improvement from 2015 to 2016 data that showed a 2% decrease.[9]

NOSOCOMIAL BLOODSTREAM INFECTIONS

The incidence of nosocomial BSIs between 1995 and 2002 was 60 cases per 10,000 hospital admissions. Intravascular devices, of which 72% were central venous catheters, were the most common predisposing factor.[32] NHSN reported between 2011 and 2014 there were 85,994 central line–associated bloodstream infection (CLABSIs) with a mortality rate of 10% to 20%.[33] In 2000, the economic cost was $40,000 per bacteremic survivor.[34]

The potential infectious breaches on a central venous catheter are demonstrated in **Fig. 3**.[33,35] Risk factors for CLABSIs include: site of insertion, multiple lumen catheters, total parenteral nutrition, low nurse-to-patient ratio, secondary infections, intravenous catheterization for longer than 3 days, inexperienced personnel, and use of stopcocks.[33] Any organism penetrating a central venous catheter can cause CLABSIs. The most common organisms are *Staphylococcus* species, Enterococci, *Candida* species, and GNB infections.[36] Drug resistance, including fluoroquinolone resistance and extended-spectrum β-lactamase-producing organisms is becoming more prevalent. Carbapenem-resistant Enterobacteriaceae pathogens comprised 7.1% of

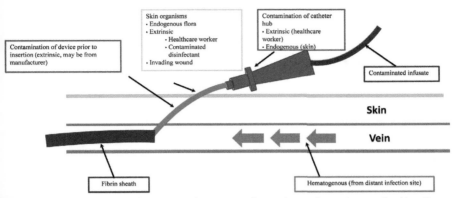

Fig. 3. Sources of infection from central venous catheter. (*Data from*: Agency for Heatlhcare Research and Quality. Appendix 3. Guidelines to Prevent Central Line-Associated Blood Stream Infections. U.S. Department of Health and Human Services. https://www.ahrq.gov/hai/clabsi-tools/appendix-3.html#s14. Updated March 2018. Accessed September 18, 2019; and Safdar N, Maki DG. The pathogenesis of catheter-related bloodstream infection with noncuffed short-term central venous catheters. *Intensive Care Med.* 2004;30(1):62-67.)

CLABSIs reported in 2014.[36] Measures to prevent CLABSIs include: stringent infection control practices, use of chlorhexidine as skin preparation before line insertion, removal of unnecessary catheters, and avoidance of femoral vein catheterization.[33,37]

Between 2008 and 2016, there was a 50% national reduction in CLABSIs as a result of collaborative efforts between national and state agencies.[9] **Fig. 4** illustrates CLABSIs standardized infection ratios calculated using 2015 and historical baseline model, and demonstrates the changes in CLABSI in US hospitals between 2006 and 2016.[9]

With data now helping guide best practices for catheter insertion and care, rates of CLABSIs reported by NHSN continue to decline. Between 2016 and 2017 there was a 9% statistically significant decrease in CLABSIs.[9]

NOSOCOMIAL SURGICAL SITE INFECTIONS

Nosocomial SSIs (NSSIs) are the most frequent unplanned cause for postoperative readmission[38] and the most common NI among surgical patients.[39] NSSIs are also the most costly HAI type.[40] NSSIs, which causes 11% of all ICU deaths,[2] are classified by the CDC to be an infection in an "incisional, organ or organ space manipulated during an operation" that occurs within 30 days of surgery or within 90 days of surgery if a prosthetic device is implanted.[41] In 2006, 80 million surgical procedures were performed in the United States of which 2% to 5% developed NSSIs.[5,40] This estimate is believed to be underreported because approximately 50% to 84% of NSSIs are evident after discharge.[2] In addition, certain techniques are used to achieve lower NSSI rates and reporting is also voluntary.[2,39] The impact of NSSIs include poorer patient outcome, increased hospital stays, and lower reimbursements to hospitals.[39] Each NSSI may cost from $1000 to $90,000 to treat. In the United States, the total annual cost of NSSIs is estimated to be $700 million.[8]

The incidence of NSSI varies from surgical procedure, surgeon, other health care providers, surgical center, and patient. Patients at highest risk for NSSIs are older in age with an emergent admission and with at least one comorbidity.[42] Approximately half of NSSIs are estimated to be preventable. Modifiable risks for SSIs include:

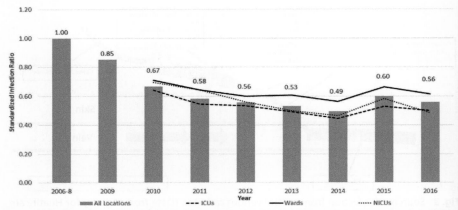

Fig. 4. Changes over time in CLABSI standardized infection ratios in US hospitals using 2006 to 2008 baseline, NHSN 2009 to 2016. NICU, neonatal ICU. (*Data from*: Centers for Disease Control and Prevention. Data Summary of HAIs in the US: Assessing Progress 2006-2016. https://www.cdc.gov/hai/data/archive/data-summary-assessing-progress.html?CDC_AA_refVal=https%3A%2F%2Fwww.cdc.gov%2Fhai%2Fsurveillance%2Fdata-reports%2Fdata-summary-assessing-progress.html.)

minimizing presurgical risk factors (smoking cessation, malnourished state), immunosuppressed state, appropriate surgical preparation, and optimizing conditions during surgery.[4,39] The CDC monitors several surgeries for NSSIs, including cardiovascular, colon, rectal, pelvic, hip, and knee procedures.[40]

NSSIs are commonly caused by bacteria or fungi invasion of the skin, soft tissue, or organ space via trauma or surgery.[43] For clean surgeries that do not involve the gastrointestinal, respiratory, or female genital tracts, gram-positive bacteria (GPB), such as SA, coagulase-negative staphylococcus, and streptococcal species from the endogenous or exogenous environment are the most common organisms cultured. For surgeries involving the gastrointestinal or female genital tracts, in addition to GPB, GNB coliforms and anaerobes need to be considered. To optimize bacterial growth, cultures should be obtained before initiating antibiotics to identify the causative organism and narrow antimicrobial coverage.

A breach in sterile technique from any health care provider can contribute to NSSIs. In the 1990s, propofol vials were reused and contaminated by anesthesia personal, which resulted in 155 patients infected across 20 states and of those four patients died. Isolated organisms included GPB, GNB, and fungi.[44]

NHSN reported an overall decrease in NSSIs from 2010 to 2014 as illustrated in **Fig. 5**.[9] Between 2016 and 2017 there was a 1% statistically significant improvement in 10 procedures but there was no improvement in abdominal hysterectomy or colon surgery SSIs.[9]

OUTBREAKS

Outbreaks of HAIs can be with a singular organism or polymicrobial and etiologies have included bacteria, fungi, viruses, and prions. A variety of reservoirs including contaminated medical equipment, such as duodenoscopes, reused injectable solutions, and health care workers have been reservoirs. Various outbreaks over the last 20 years are listed in **Tables 1** and **2**.[4,45–55] Methods to prevent and control outbreaks

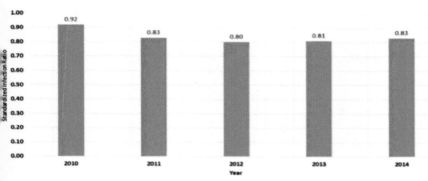

Fig. 5. Changes over time in SSI after any of 10 surgical care improvement project procedures in US hospitals using 2006 to 2008 baseline, NHSN 2010 to 2014. (*Data from:* Centers for Disease Control and Prevention. Data Summary of HAIs in the US: Assessing Progress 006-2016. https://www.cdc.gov/hai/data/archive/data-summary-assessing-progress.html?CDC_AA_refVal=https%3A%2F%2Fwww.cdc.gov%2Fhai%2Fsurveillance%2Fdata-reports%2Fdata-summary-assessing-progress.html. Updated December 5, 2017. Accessed September 18, 2019.)

Table 1
Summary of nosocomial outbreaks

Year	Organism	Location	Number of Cases	Number of Deaths	Source
2016	*Candida auris*	ICU in United Kingdom	70	0	Reusable axillary temperature probes[45]
2016	*Bulkholderia cepacia*	59 long-term and rehabilitation facilities[a]	163	9	0.9% sodium chloride IV flush by nurse assistant[46]
2016	Polymicrobial[b]	Quebec, Canada	9	0	Suboptimal cavitron ultrasonic surgical aspirator cleaning used in craniotomy/craniectomy.[54]
2014	Carbapenemase-resistant Enterobacteriaciae	UCLA	9	2	Duodenoscopes[47]
2012–2013	*Exserohilum rostratum*	25 states	753	64	New England Compounding Center[48] Preservative-free MPA

Abbreviations: IV, intravenous; MPA, methylprednisolone acetate; UCLA, University of California, Los Angeles.
a Delaware, Maryland, New Jersey, and Pennsylvania.
b *Opionibacterium acnes* (n = 5), *Staphylococcus aureus* (n = 2), *Streptococcus agalactiae* (n = l), *Enterococcus faecalis* (n = l), *Bacteroides fragilis* (n = l), polymicrobial (n = 2).

Table 2
Summary of nosocomial outbreaks

Year	Organism	Location	Number of Cases	Number of Deaths	Source
2011	*Klebsiella pneumoniae* carbapenemases	US NIHCC-ICU[a]	18	11	Inanimate objects Ventilators Hospital equipment[49]
2008	MRSA and MSSA (FusR)	United Kingdom[b]	19		MSSA (FusR) colonized health care worker with psoriasis[50]
2008	HCV	New York[c]	657 exposed, 3 seroconverted	0	Hemodialysis machine[51]
2006–2007	HCV and HBV	New York colonoscopy clinic	50,000 exposed, 6 HBV, 6 HCV, 1 HBV + HCV	0	Reused syringes administering propofol vials by 1 anesthesiologist[52]
1998	HCV	Florida	3	0	Reused multisaline vials[55]
1998	Pseudomonas UTI	Pediatric surgical ICU	14	0	Tap water[53]

Abbreviations: HBV, hepatitis B virus; HCV, hepatitis C virus; MRSA, methicillin-resistant *Staphylococcus aureus*; MSSA, methicillin-sensitive *Staphylococcus aureus*; UTI, urinary tract infection.
[a] US National Institutes of Health Clinical Center-ICU.
[b] Nottingham University Hospital, Nottingham, UK.
[c] New York Outpatient Hemodialysis Center.

include strict handwashing, proper cleaning of equipment, isolation of patients colonized with MDROs, and antimicrobial stewardship.[56]

Staphylococcus aureus

SA is a highly adaptable and virulent organism and is among the most common causes of NIs, including CLABSI, infective endocarditis, HCAP, skin and soft tissue infections, and SSIs.[57] Approximately 30% of people are asymptomatic carriers in the back of their noses.[58] Exogenous spread of SA occurs by direct contact with an infected wound or from contaminated health care workers' hands.[59]

SA was initially treated with penicillin; however, resistance occurred in hospitals shortly after its regular use.[60–62] To overcome SA's penicillin resistance, methicillin, a semisynthetic penicillin, was introduced in 1959, but methicillin-resistant SA (MRSA) emerged shortly thereafter in 1961. The first reported US outbreak of hospital-acquired MRSA infection occurred in 1963.[60,61] Over time, the rate of hospital-acquired MRSA in US hospitals increased from 4% in the 1980s to 50% by the late 1990s.[59,60] However, community-acquired MRSA infections were sporadic in nature until the 1990s, when community-acquired MRSA infections by a new strain (USA 300 clone) were reported among children,[63] team members,[64,65] correctional facilities,[66] day care centers,[67] and military personnel.[68,69] Community-acquired MRSA strains subsequently integrated in nosocomial settings.[60] By 2013, the CDC deemed MRSA to be a serious threat to the world.[16] Risk factors for MRSA infection include immunocompromised state, prosthetic or invasive devices, residing in the ICU, MRSA self-colonization, and open wounds.[70]

By 2011, invasive MRSA infections are estimated to have caused 80,000 US cases and 11,000 annual deaths.[16] Between 2005 and 2014, the overall incidence of hospital-acquired MRSA infections declined by 65%, contributing to interventions designed to decrease transmission and reduce the risk of device- and procedure-associated infections.[59,71] CDC's most recent report on HAIs demonstrates an 8% statistically significant reduction in MRSA bacteremia between 2016 and 2017.[7]

Since its introduction in 1972, vancomycin became the only reliable agent against MRSA. Vancomycin-intermediate SA (minimum inhibitory concentration of 4–8 μg mL^{-1}), first reported in 1997, and vancomycin-resistant S aureus, first described in Japan in 1996,[72] both entered the United States in 2002[73] and have become emerging threats to the world.[74] Risk factors for vancomycin-resistant S aureus include MRSA and vancomycin-resistant enterococci colonization, MRSA bacteremia with central line or prosthesis, chronic medical conditions (diabetes, dialysis), prolonged vancomycin use, and chronic skin ulcers.[75,76]

Hepatitis C Virus

Nosocomial hepatitis C virus (HCV) infection was historically most commonly transmitted via hemodialysis (HD), blood transfusions, and needle stick injuries. However there have been reports of other mechanisms of transmission including unsafe injection practices with reused contaminated medications, inadequate cleaning of reusable contaminated equipment, and colonoscopy with biopsies.[52]

Since the advent of blood donation screening for HCV in 1990, the risk of HCV in blood transfusion has been nearly eliminated. Before 1990, 10% of transfusion recipients acquired HCV.[77] Currently, HD still poses the highest risk, especially in-hospital HD. Periodic screening is recommended for HD patients because in some parts of the United States, almost 10% of HD patients become seropositive. There are several factors that increase a patient's risk during HD, including the prevalence of HCV patients in the dialysis units and length of time on HD.

Clostridium difficile Infection

The bacteria *C difficile* was first isolated from the stool of a healthy infant in 1935; however, pseudomembranous colitis was first described in 1893. In 1978, following the introduction of broad-spectrum antibiotics in the 1960s and 1970s, *C difficile* was determined to be the organism responsible for most cases of antibiotic-associated diarrhea and pseudomembranous colitis.[78]

A new *C difficile* strain highly resistant to clindamycin, which was discovered between 1989 and 1992, was identified to have caused *C difficile* infectious (CDIs) outbreaks in four unrelated US hospitals.[79] By the early 2000s several US and Canadian institutions noted an increasing incidence and severity of CDIs among patients exposed to fluoroquinolones and cephalosporins.[80–82] Between 2000 and 2003 *C difficile* isolates collected from eight health care facilities in six states discovered a highly transmissible, more resistant and virulent strain termed BI/NAP1/027,[83] which produced about 10-fold more toxin A and 23-fold more toxin B than previous strains.[84,85] Higher relapse rates also occurred.[86]

Currently, CDIs cause HAIs worldwide and more than a million cases per year in the United States.[87] Between 10% and 30% of patients develop at least one recurrent CDI after the first diagnosis. The risk of recurrence increases with each successive episode.[88,89] Recurrent CDI is associated with a 33% increased risk of mortality at 180 days relative to patients who do not develop a recurrence.[89] In 2013, the CDC assigned CDI as an urgent threat to the world.[16]

Patients who have failed multiple antibiotic courses for recurrent CDI pose a particular challenge. Fecal microbiota transplantation (FMT) for recurrent CDI has an estimated success rate of 77% to 100% depending on the route of instillation of feces.[89] Therefore, 2018 guidelines recommended FMT for patients with multiple recurrences of CDI who have failed appropriate antibiotic courses.[89]

More recent data, however, demonstrate FMT may not be as effective. A recent meta-analysis of 13 trials showed that studies for recurrent CDI reported higher resolution rates than studies that used FMT for recurrent and refractory CDI. There was a lower efficacy for FMT in patients who have refractory disease compared with standard-of-care antibiotics.[90]

FMT also have safety concerns because the microbiota is associated with a host of unknown chronic medical conditions, including diabetes mellitus, obesity, cancer, and autoimmune disorders. In addition, infectious complications attributed to FMT have included norovirus gastroenteritis, cytomegalovirus, and bacteremias with *Escherichia coli*, *Proteus mirabilis*, *Citrobacter koseri*, and *Enterococcus faecium*.[91] Recently, the Food and Drug Administration issued a warning, after two patients developed extended-spectrum β-lactamase-producing *E coli* infections and one of those patients died.[92] Because of these conflicting reports, more data are needed to determine the overall safety and efficacy of FMT in CDI.

SUMMARY

HAIs continue to be a major factor in morbidity and mortality, rising health care costs, and the prevalence of drug-resistant organisms. However, most NIs are preventable and effective strategies implemented by the CDC-NHSN in conjunction with health care facilities have demonstrated monitoring and interventions are productive in educing HAIs to decrease morbidity and mortality, save billions of health care dollars, nd reduce the spread of MDROs.

DISCLOSURE

-Y. Liu writes infectious disease content for AMPSAA Web site; J.K. Dickter has othing to report.

REFERENCES

1. Haque M, Sartelli M, McKimm J, et al. Health care-associated infections: an overview. Infect Drug Resist 2018;11:2321–33.
2. Klevens RM, Edwards JR, Richards CL Jr, et al. Estimating health care-associated infections and deaths in U.S. hospitals, 2002. Public Health Rep 2007;122(2):160–6.
3. Siegel JD, Rhinehart E, Jackson M, et al. 2007 guideline for isolation precautions: preventing transmission of infectious agents in healthcare settings 2018. Available at: https://www.cdc.gov/infectioncontrol/guidelines/isolation/index.html. Accessed September 18, 2019.
4. Sheitoyan-Pesant C, Alarie I, Grenier O, et al. Investigation of an outbreak of surgical site infections following craniotomies, associated with a cavitron ultrasonic surgical aspirator. Open Forum Infect Dis 2016;3(suppl_1):1445.
5. Khan HA, Baig FK, Mehboob R. Nosocomial infections: epidemiology, prevention, control and surveillance. Asian Pac J Trop Biomed 2017;7(5):478–82.
6. Peleg AY, Hooper DC. Hospital-acquired infections due to gram-negative bacteria. N Engl J Med 2010;362(19):1804–13.
7. Centers for Disease Control and Prevention. Current HAI progress report 2017. Available at: https://www.cdc.gov/hai/data/portal/progress-report.html. Accessed September 18, 2019.
8. Scott RD. The direct medical costs of healthcare-associated infections in U.S. hospitals and the benefits of prevention. In: National Center for Preparedness D, Control of Infectious Diseases. Division of Healthcare Quality P, editors. Division of Healthcare Quality Promotion National Center for Preparedness, Detection, and Control of Infectious Diseases, Centers for Disease Control and Prevention; 2009. Available at: https://www.cdc.gov/HAI/pdfs/hai/scott_costpaper.pdf. Accessed September 18, 2019.
9. Centers for Disease Control and Prevention. Data summary of HAIs in the US: assessing progress 2006-2016. 2017. Available at: https://www.cdc.gov/hai/data/archive/data-summary-assessing-progress.html?CDC_AA_refVal=https%3A%2F%2Fwww.cdc.gov%2Fhai%2Fsurveillance%2Fdata-reports%2Fdata-summary-assessing-progress.html. Accessed September 18, 2019.
10. Centers for Disease Control and Prevention. About NHSN 2019. Available at: https://www.cdc.gov/nhsn/about-nhsn/index.html. Accessed September 19, 2019.
11. Tokars JI, Richards C, Andrus M, et al. The changing face of surveillance for health care-associated infections. Clin Infect Dis 2004;39(9):1347–52.
12. Public health focus: surveillance, prevention, and control of nosocomial infections. MMWR Morb Mortal Wkly Rep 1992;41(42):783–7.
13. Centers for Disease Control and Prevention. Catheter-associated urinary tract infections (CAUTI). 2015. Available at: https://www.cdc.gov/hai/ca_uti/uti.html. Accessed September 18, 2019.

14. Elliott C, Justiz-Vaillant A. Nosocomial infections: a 360-degree review. Int Bio Biomed J 2018;4(2):72–81.

15. Gharbi M, Drysdale JH, Lishman H, et al. Antibiotic management of urinary trac infection in elderly patients in primary care and its association with bloodstream infections and all-cause mortality: population based cohort study. BMJ 2019;364 l525.

16. Centers for Disease Control and Prevention. Antibiotic resistance threats in the United States, 2013 2013. Available at: https://www.cdc.gov/drugresistance pdf/ar-threats-2013-508.pdf. Accessed September 18, 2019.

17. Bou G, Cervero G, Dominguez MA, et al. Characterization of a nosocomia outbreak caused by a multiresistant *Acinetobacter baumannii* strain with a carbapenem-hydrolyzing enzyme: high-level carbapenem resistance in *A. baumannii* is not due solely to the presence of beta-lactamases. J Clin Micro biol 2000;38(9):3299–305.

18. Liu J, Du SX, Zhang JN, et al. Spreading of extended-spectrum beta-lactamase producing *Escherichia coli* ST131 and *Klebsiella pneumoniae* ST11 in patients with pneumonia: a molecular epidemiological study. Chin Med J (Engl) 2019 132(16):1894–902.

19. Mitchell BG, Russo PL, Cheng AC, et al. Strategies to reduce non-ventilator associated hospital-acquired pneumonia: a systematic review. Infect Dis Health 2019;24(4):229–39.

20. Russo PL, Stewardson AJ, Cheng AC, et al. The prevalence of healthcare asso ciated infections among adult inpatients at nineteen large Australian acute-care public hospitals: a point prevalence survey. Antimicrob Resist Infect Contro 2019;8:114.

21. Vincent JL, Rello J, Marshall J, et al. International study of the prevalence and out comes of infection in intensive care units. JAMA 2009;302(21):2323–9.

22. Stone PW, Hedblom EC, Murphy DM, et al. The economic impact of infection con trol: making the business case for increased infection control resources. Am J Infect Control 2005;33(9):542–7.

23. Kalil AC, Metersky ML, Klompas M, et al. Management of adults with hospital acquired and ventilator-associated pneumonia: 2016 Clinical Practice Guidelines by the Infectious Diseases Society of America and the American Thoracic Soci ety. Clin Infect Dis 2016;63(5):e61–111.

24. Iacovelli V, Gaziev G, Topazio L, et al. Nosocomial urinary tract infections: a re view. Urologia 2014;81(4):222–7.

25. Meddings J, Saint S, Fowler KE, et al. The Ann Arbor criteria for appropriate uri nary catheter use in hospitalized medical patients: results obtained by using the RAND/UCLA appropriateness method. Ann Intern Med 2015;162(9 Suppl) S1–34.

26. Hooton TM, Bradley SF, Cardenas DD, et al. Diagnosis, prevention, and treatment of catheter-associated urinary tract infection in adults: 2009 International Clinical Practice Guidelines from the Infectious Diseases Society of America. Clin Infect Dis 2010;50(5):625–63.

27. Delcaru C, Alexandru I, Podgoreanu P, et al. Microbial biofilms in urinary tract in fections and prostatitis: etiology, pathogenicity, and combating strategies. Path ogens 2016;5(4):65.

28. Nicolle LE. Health care–acquired urinary tract infection: the problem and solu tions. Agency for Healthcare Research and Quality. Patient Safety Network Web site. 2008. Available at: https://psnet.ahrq.gov/perspectives/perspective/

68/Health-CareAcquired-Urinary-Tract-Infection-The-Problem-and-Solutions. Accessed September 18, 2019.

29. Guidelines for prevention of nosocomial pneumonia. Centers for Disease Control and Prevention. MMWR Recomm Rep 1997;46(Rr-1):1–79.

30. Esperatti M, Ferrer M, Giunta V, et al. Validation of predictors of adverse outcomes in hospital-acquired pneumonia in the ICU. Crit Care Med 2013;41(9): 2151–61.

31. Huxley EJ, Viroslav J, Gray WR, et al. Pharyngeal aspiration in normal adults and patients with depressed consciousness. Am J Med 1978;64(4):564–8.

32. Wisplinghoff H, Bischoff T, Tallent SM, et al. Nosocomial bloodstream infections in US hospitals: analysis of 24,179 cases from a prospective nationwide surveillance study. Clin Infect Dis 2004;39(3):309–17.

33. Agency for Heatlhcare Research and Quality. Appendix 3. Guidelines to prevent central line-associated blood stream infections. U.S. Department of Health and Human Services; 2018. Available at: https://www.ahrq.gov/hai/clabsi-tools/appendix-3.html#s14. Accessed September 18, 2019.

34. Centers for Disease Control and Prevention. Central line-associated bloodstream infection - (CLABSI). 2010. Available at: https://www.cdc.gov/hai/bsi/bsi.html. Accessed September 18, 2019.

35. Safdar N, Maki DG. The pathogenesis of catheter-related bloodstream infection with noncuffed short-term central venous catheters. Intensive Care Med 2004; 30(1):62–7.

36. Weiner LM, Webb AK, Limbago B, et al. Antimicrobial-resistant pathogens associated with healthcare-associated infections: summary of data reported to the National Healthcare Safety Network at the Centers for Disease Control and Prevention, 2011-2014. Infect Control Hosp Epidemiol 2016;37(11):1288–301.

37. O'Grady NP, Alexander M, Burns LA, et al. Guidelines for the prevention of intravascular catheter-related infections. Clin Infect Dis 2011;52(9):e162–93.

38. Merkow RP, Ju MH, Chung JW, et al. Underlying reasons associated with hospital readmission following surgery in the United States. JAMA 2015;313(5):483–95.

39. Mellinghoff SC, Vehreschild JJ, Liss BJ, et al. Epidemiology of surgical site infections with *Staphylococcus aureus* in Europe: protocol for a retrospective, multicenter study. JMIR Res Protoc 2018;7(3):e63.

40. Centers for Disease Control and Prevention. Surgical site infection (SSI) event. In: Procedure-associated module - SSI. Atlanta (GA): Centers for Disease Control and Prevention; 2019. Available at: https://www.cdc.gov/nhsn/pdfs/pscManual/9pscSSIcurrent.pdf. Accessed September 18, 2019.

41. Nichols RL. Preventing surgical site infections: a surgeon's perspective. Emerg Infect Dis 2001;7(2):220–4.

42. Stulberg JJ, Delaney CP, Neuhauser DV, et al. Adherence to surgical care improvement project measures and the association with postoperative infections. JAMA 2010;303(24):2479–85.

43. Berrios-Torres SI, Umscheid CA, Bratzler DW, et al. Centers for Disease Control and Prevention Guideline for the Prevention of Surgical Site Infection, 2017. JAMA Surg 2017;152(8):784–91.

44. Bennett SN, McNeil MM, Bland LA, et al. Postoperative infections traced to contamination of an intravenous anesthetic, propofol. N Engl J Med 1995; 333(3):147–54.

45. Eyre DW, Sheppard AE, Madder H, et al. A *Candida auris* outbreak and its control in an intensive care setting. N Engl J Med 2018;379(14):1322–31.

46. Brooks RB, Mitchell PK, Miller JR, et al. Multistate outbreak of *Burkholderia cepacia* complex bloodstream infections after exposure to contaminated saline flush syringes—United States, 2016-2017. Clin Infect Dis 2018;69(3):445–9.

47. Humphries RM, Yang S, Kim S, et al. Duodenoscope-related outbreak of a carbapenem-resistant *Klebsiella pneumoniae* identified using advanced molecular diagnostics. Clin Infect Dis 2017;65(7):1159–66.

48. Smith RM, Derado G, Wise M, et al. Estimated deaths and illnesses averted during fungal meningitis outbreak associated with contaminated steroid injections, United States, 2012-2013. Emerg Infect Dis 2015;21(6):933–40.

49. Snitkin ES, Zelazny AM, Thomas PJ, et al. Tracking a hospital outbreak of carbapenem-resistant *Klebsiella pneumoniae* with whole-genome sequencing. Sci Transl Med 2012;4(148) [art no. 148ra116].

50. Crusz SA, Yates C, Holden S, et al. Prolonged outbreak of *Staphylococcus aureus* surgical site infection traced to a healthcare worker with psoriasis. J Hosp Infect 2014;86(1):42–6.

51. Hepatitis C virus transmission at an outpatient hemodialysis unit—New York, 2001-2008. MMWR Morb Mortal Wkly Rep 2009;58(8):189–94.

52. Gutelius B, Perz JF, Parker MM, et al. Multiple clusters of hepatitis virus infections associated with anesthesia for outpatient endoscopy procedures. Gastroenterology 2010;139(1):163–70.

53. Ferroni A, Nguyen L, Pron B, et al. Outbreak of nosocomial urinary tract infections due to *Pseudomonas aeruginosa* in a paediatric surgical unit associated with tap-water contamination. J Hosp Infect 1998;39(4):301–7.

54. Sheitoyan-Pesant C, Alarie I, Grenier O, etal. Investigation of an Outbreak of Surgical Site Infections Following Craniotomies, Associated with a Cavitron Ultrasonic Surgical Aspirator. Open Forum Infectious Diseases 2016;3:1445.

55. Krause G, Trepka M, Whisenhunt R, et al. Nosocomial Transmission of Hepatitis C Virus Associated With the Use of Multidose Saline Vials. Infect Control Hosp Epidemiol 2003 Feb;24(2):122–7.

56. Centers for Disease Control and Prevention. National Center for Emerging and Zoonotic Infectious Diseases (NCEZID), Division of Healthcare Quality Promotion (DHQP). Guidelines & Guidance Library. 2019. Available at: https://www.cdc.gov/infectioncontrol/guidelines/index.html. Accessed September 18, 2019.

57. Centers for Disease Control and Prevention. *Staphylococcus aureus* in healthcare settings. Available at: https://www.cdc.gov/hai/organisms/staph.html. Accessed September 18, 2019.

58. Wertheim HF, Melles DC, Vos MC, et al. The role of nasal carriage in *Staphylococcus aureus* infections. Lancet Infect Dis 2005;5(12):751–62.

59. Centers for Disease Control and Prevention. Methicillin-resistant *Staphylococcus aureus* (MRSA). 2019. Available at: https://www.cdc.gov/mrsa/healthcare/index.html. Accessed September 18, 2019.

60. Sampathkumar P. Methicillin-resistant *Staphylococcus aureus*: the latest health scare. Mayo Clin Proc 2007;82(12):1463–7.

61. Stryjewski ME, Corey GR. Methicillin-resistant *Staphylococcus aureus*: an evolving pathogen. Clin Infect Dis 2014;58(Suppl 1):S10–9.

62. Stewart GT, Holt RJ. Evolution of natural resistance to the newer penicillins. Br Med J 1963;1(5326):308–11.

63. Four pediatric deaths from community-acquired methicillin-resistant *Staphylococcus aureus*—Minnesota and North Dakota, 1997-1999. MMWR Morb Mortal Wkly Rep 1999;48(32):707–10.

4. Kazakova SV, Hageman JC, Matava M, et al. A clone of methicillin-resistant *Staphylococcus aureus* among professional football players. N Engl J Med 2005;352(5):468–75.

5. Lindenmayer JM, Schoenfeld S, O'Grady R, et al. Methicillin-resistant *Staphylococcus aureus* in a high school wrestling team and the surrounding community. Arch Intern Med 1998;158(8):895–9.

6. Methicillin-resistant *Staphylococcus aureus* infections in correctional facilities— Georgia, California, and Texas, 2001-2003. MMWR Morb Mortal Wkly Rep 2003;52(41):992–6.

7. Jensen JU, Jensen ET, Larsen AR, et al. Control of a methicillin-resistant *Staphylococcus aureus* (MRSA) outbreak in a day-care institution. J Hosp Infect 2006; 63(1):84–92.

8. Beilman GJ, Sandifer G, Skarda D, et al. Emerging infections with community-associated methicillin-resistant *Staphylococcus aureus* in outpatients at an Army community hospital. Surg Infect (Larchmt) 2005;6(1):87–92.

9. Pagac BB, Reiland RW, Bolesh DT, et al. Skin lesions in barracks: consider community-acquired methicillin-resistant *Staphylococcus aureus* infection instead of spider bites. Mil Med 2006;171(9):830–2.

0. Leibler JH, Leon C, Cardoso LJP, et al. Prevalence and risk factors for MRSA nasal colonization among persons experiencing homelessness in Boston, MA. J Med Microbiol 2017;66(8):1183–8.

1. Centers for Disease Control and Prevention. Strategies to prevent hospital-onset *Staphylococcus aureus* bloodstream infections in acute care facilities. 2019. Available at: https://www.cdc.gov/hai/prevent/staph-prevention-strategies.html. Accessed September 18, 2019.

2. Hiramatsu K, Hanaki H, Ino T, et al. Methicillin-resistant *Staphylococcus aureus* clinical strain with reduced vancomycin susceptibility. J Antimicrob Chemother 1997;40(1):135–6.

3. Centers for Disease Control and Prevention (CDC). Vancomycin-resistant *Staphylococcus aureus*—Pennsylvania, 2002. MMWR Morb Mortal Wkly Rep 2002; 51(40):902.

4. Foster TJ. Antibiotic resistance in *Staphylococcus aureus*. Current status and future prospects. FEMS Microbiol Rev 2017;41(3):430–49.

5. Virginia Department of Health. VISA/VRSA infections. 2018. Available at: http://www.vdh.virginia.gov/epidemiology/epidemiology-fact-sheets/vancomycin-intermediate-staphylococcus-aureus-visa-and-vancomycin-resistant-staphylo-coccus-aureus-vrsa-infections/. Accessed September 18, 2019.

6. Pennsylvania Department of Health. Vancomycin-resistant and vancomycin-intermediate *Staphylococcus aureus* (VRSA AND VISA) fact sheet. 2017. Available at: https://www.health.pa.gov/topics/Documents/Diseases%20and%20Conditions/Vancomycin_resistant%20and%20Vancomycin_intermediate%20Staphylococcus %20aureus%20.pdf. Accessed September 18, 2019.

7. Fischer GE, Schaefer MK, Labus BJ, et al. Hepatitis C virus infections from unsafe injection practices at an endoscopy clinic in Las Vegas, Nevada, 2007-2008. Clin Infect Dis 2010;51(3):267–73.

8. Bartlett JG, Chang TW, Gurwith M, et al. Antibiotic-associated pseudomembranous colitis due to toxin-producing clostridia. N Engl J Med 1978;298(10):531–4.

9. Johnson S, Samore MH, Farrow KA, et al. Epidemics of diarrhea caused by a clindamycin-resistant strain of *Clostridium difficile* in four hospitals. N Engl J Med 1999;341(22):1645–51.

80. Loo VG, Poirier L, Miller MA, et al. A predominantly clonal multi-institutional outbreak of *Clostridium difficile*-associated diarrhea with high morbidity and mortality. N Engl J Med 2005;353(23):2442–9.

81. Muto CA, Pokrywka M, Shutt K, et al. A large outbreak of *Clostridium difficile* associated disease with an unexpected proportion of deaths and colectomies at a teaching hospital following increased fluoroquinolone use. Infect Control Hosp Epidemiol 2005;26(3):273–80.

82. Pepin J, Valiquette L, Alary ME, et al. *Clostridium difficile*-associated diarrhea in a region of Quebec from 1991 to 2003: a changing pattern of disease severity. CMAJ 2004;171(5):466–72.

83. McDonald LC, Killgore GE, Thompson A, et al. An epidemic, toxin gene-variant strain of *Clostridium difficile*. N Engl J Med 2005;353(23):2433–41.

84. Kelly CP, LaMont JT. *Clostridium difficile*: more difficult than ever. N Engl J Med 2008;359(18):1932–40.

85. Warny M, Pepin J, Fang A, et al. Toxin production by an emerging strain of *Clostridium difficile* associated with outbreaks of severe disease in North America and Europe. Lancet 2005;366(9491):1079–84.

86. Bartlett JG. Narrative review: the new epidemic of *Clostridium difficile*-associated enteric disease. Ann Intern Med 2006;145(10):758–64.

87. Gorbach SL, Bartlett JG. Contributions to the discovery of *Clostridium difficile* antibiotic-associated diarrhea. Clin Infect Dis 2014;59(suppl_2):S66–70.

88. Gough E, Shaikh H, Manges AR. Systematic review of intestinal microbiota transplantation (fecal bacteriotherapy) for recurrent *Clostridium difficile* infection. Clin Infect Dis 2011;53(10):994–1002.

89. McDonald LC, Gerding DN, Johnson S, et al. Clinical practice guidelines for *Clostridium difficile* infection in adults and children: 2017 update by the Infectious Diseases Society of America (IDSA) and Society for Healthcare Epidemiology of America (SHEA). Clin Infect Dis 2018;66(7):987–94.

90. Tariq R, Pardi DS, Bartlett MG, et al. Low cure rates in controlled trials of fecal microbiota transplantation for recurrent *Clostridium difficile* infection: a systematic review and meta-analysis. Clin Infect Dis 2019;68(8):1351–8.

91. Wang S, Xu M, Wang W, et al. Systematic review: adverse events of fecal microbiota transplantation. PLoS One 2016;11(8):e0161174.

92. Food and Drug Administration (FDA). Important safety alert regarding use of fecal microbiota for transplantation and risk of serious adverse reactions due to transmission of multi-drug resistant organisms 2019. Available at: https://www.fda.gov/vaccines-blood-biologics/safety-availability-biologics/important-safety-alert-regarding-use-fecal-microbiota-transplantation-and-risk-serious-adverse. Accessed September 18, 2019.

Duodenoscope as a Vector for Transmission

Jennifer T. Higa, MD[a],*, Andrew S. Ross, MD[b]

KEYWORDS

- Cross-contamination • Infection control • Duodenoscopes
- Linear echoendoscopes • Endoscopic retrograde cholangiopancreatography
- High-level disinfection • Multidrug resistant organisms

KEY POINTS

- Advancements in endoscope technology and design are needed to ensure greater safety for patients undergoing ERCP and endoscopic ultrasound.
- Interim solutions have emerged to include enhanced cleaning methods, quality metrics and redundancy built into the reprocessing procedures, exhaustive informed consent, and routine maintenance of endoscopes.
- Such protective factors may have mitigated risk but even in combination remains an unlikely panacea.
- Staff training and competency must also be prioritized; however, other implementable and wholly important measures include skill task alignment, ergonomic workspace optimization, and a feedback process for all levels of staff to report system problems in a nonthreatening manner.
- An obvious long-term solution is a design change eliminating the current elevator mechanism; however, even with novel designs, such as the removable duodenoscope cap or even fully disposable instruments, the feasibility of use, cost effectiveness, and long-term efficacy of these changes is yet to be determined.

INTRODUCTION

In 2012, multiple reports from Europe and the United States described outbreaks of infection from multidrug-resistant organisms (MDRO) in patients who had undergone endoscopic retrograde cholangiopancreatography (ERCP). In some cases, these infections resulted in significant injury and death and almost always occurred without obvious breaches in standard high-level disinfection (HLD) protocols. Individual, site-based investigation into these outbreaks incriminated the complex design of the duodenoscope, more specifically that the cantilevered elevator mechanism was prone to retention of bioburden serving as the source of patient cross-contamination.[1]

[a] Division of Gastroenterology, Fox Chase Cancer Center, 333 Cottman Avenue, P3179, Philadelphia, PA 19111, USA; [b] Division of Gastroenterology, Virginia Mason Medical Center, 1100 Ninth Avenue, C3GAS, Seattle, WA 98101, USA
* Corresponding author.
E-mail address: Jennifer.higa@fccc.edu

Gastrointest Endoscopy Clin N Am 30 (2020) 653–663
https://doi.org/10.1016/j.giec.2020.05.002   giendo.theclinics.com
1052-5157/20/© 2020 Elsevier Inc. All rights reserved.

Duodenoscope-associated patient cross-contamination is now understood to be a multifactorial problem related to issues with device design, maintenance, and function, with additional risk incurred from an HLD process that lacks quality controls. Curvilinear array echoendoscopes have also been implicated given a similarly complex design.

Extensive efforts by endoscopy centers, industry, and regulatory bodies are underway to optimize the safety of these vital instruments. ERCP and endoscopic ultrasound remain critical diagnostic and therapeutic platforms for the minimally invasive treatment of pancreaticobiliary disease. Examinations using these instruments are cornerstones in the work-up and management of benign and malignant conditions affecting the gastrointestinal tract. In this article, we address the culpability of these scopes as a vector of transmission and review the historical context of recent endoscope-related outbreaks, technical aspects of scope design contributing to this risk, and measures taken to overcome these shortcomings with areas of ongoing research.

THE ELEVATOR AND ITS ROLE IN SCOPE-RELATED INFECTIONS: A HISTORICAL BACKGROUND

Since 2012 there have been dozens of reported duodenoscope-related outbreaks of infections from MDRO in patients undergoing ERCP.[1-5] Although infectious complications from endogenous bacteria are a known procedural risk, the transmission of exogenous bacteria between patients implies a defect in HLD. Although endoscope-associated patient cross-contamination has been well documented in the medical literature,[6-9] before 2012, these reports had always been associated with a major, systemic breach in HLD. The recent infections, however, occurred despite apparent site compliance with manufacturer-recommended reprocessing techniques. Outbreak sites were typically large, well-resourced medical centers performing higher volume endoscopy and, in some cases, equipped to detect trends in infection-related complication rates.

Investigators from the Erasmus Hospital in the Netherlands were among the first to report this phenomenon, describing infections from a VIM-2-producing *Pseudomonas aeruginosa* following the introduction of the TJF-Q180V duodenoscope developed by the Olympus Corporation (Tokyo, Japan) in 2010.[5] Thirty patients were infected, with 22 of these cases singularly attributed to a newly designed duodenoscope with fixed cap. An exhaustive investigation including scope dissection with electron microscopy resulted in withdrawal of the culprit duodenoscope from use with return to baseline rates of infectious complications.

The first US-based outbreaks occurred in 2012 with a total of 19 reported outbreaks to date.[10] All three duodenoscope manufacturers have been implicated.[5,11] Consistent with the European outbreaks, the US-based cases occurred in high-volume centers without identifiable major lapses in scope reprocessing. Initial investigation of these outbreaks was individually driven by the affected medical centers. Many of the US-based cases were characterized by unique antibiotic resistance patterns and the clonality of each MDRO proven using pulsed-gel electrophoresis.[1,3,4,12] Often, culprit endoscopes were identified in each outbreak.

Subsequent efforts were made by various outbreak sites, in addition to industry and federal regulatory bodies, to characterize the HLD defect rate for duodenoscopes. One center documented a 1.9% HLD defect rate over 1-year period, for 1500 consecutive duodenoscope cultures.[12] Another center that implemented ethylene oxide (EtO) sterilization after an outbreak of carbapenem-resistant Enterobacteriaceae infections published a scope-positive culture rate of 1.2% over an 18-month period with monthly

ultures for 589 procedures.[13] Independent risk factors for MDRO transmission have
een identified to include those patients with biliary stent placement during ERCP
odds ratio, 3.62; 95% confidence interval, 1.12–11.67) and inpatient status (odds ra-
o, 3.74; 95% confidence interval, 1.15–12.12).[14] A diagnosis of cholangiocarcinoma
was also associated with increased risk. The Food and Drug Administration (FDA) sub-
equently required each manufacturer to conduct postmarket surveillance studies to
urther understand whether their instructions for use for duodenoscope HLD were
ffective in a real-world clinical setting. At the last interim analysis, the results of these
tudies suggested an HLD defect rate up to 3.6% and 5.4%, for low- and high-
oncern organisms, respectively.[15]

NDOSCOPE DESIGN
Duodenoscope

since the first ERCP performed in 1968, the duodenoscope has evolved from a semi-
eliable, side-viewing instrument to a therapeutic workhorse available in most medical
enters.[16] Modern duodenoscopes are side-viewing endoscopes equipped with an
elevator to facilitate cannulation pancreaticobiliary cannulation, and provide leverage
or instruments through a large working channel (4.2 mm, 4.8 mm) in therapeutic duodenoscopes. Three different endoscope manufacturers distribute these instruments in
he United States.

Linear Array Echoendoscope

Curvilinear array echoendoscopes were first introduced in 1991 by Pentax Corpora-
ion (FG-32, Tokyo, Japan)[17] followed by models introduced from Fujinon (EG-
30UT, Saitama, Japan) and Olympus (GF-UCT180/UCT260). Conventionally these
scopes are oblique viewing but there are also some forward-viewing models. The
modern iterations of these scopes have therapeutic working channels 3.7 to
.8 mm in diameter, and an elevator to assist needle guidance and improve maneuver-
bility of accessories.

Factors that Increase Risk

The elevator channel of these endoscopes predispose to contamination primarily
because of insufficient manual cleaning from limited access to the recessed space
behind the elevator.[18,19]

Working channels (air, water, biopsy) are challenging to clean because of a long nar-
ow caliber, but identical to other nonelevator based scopes. These channels harbor a
isk for retention of bioburden especially if channels are damaged with surface defects
and are ineffectively cleaned, two conditions that facilitate biofilm formation.[20–22]

Microbial accumulation in an impenetrable and polysaccharide matrix is commonly
eferred to as biofilm. Manual cleaning and other mechanical reprocessing methods
are more effective than standard chemical methods at physically dislodging these
adherent colonies.[23] The importance of manual cleaning was emphasized with the
elease of a manufacturer mandated manual cleaning brush, which was intended to
better address the elevator recess.[24]

OVERCOMING STANDARD ENDOSOCOPE DESIGN IN THE ERA OF MULTIDRUG RESISTANT ORGANISMS
High-Level Disinfection

n 1968, the Spaulding classification deemed flexible endoscopes semicritical instruments, requiring that they meet the standards of HLD with demonstrated 6-log10

reduction in bioburden to minimize risk of transmission of infectious pathogens.[25] HL is defined as the elimination of greater than 99% of pathogenic organisms. This is monumental task that must be performed effectively and with reproducible results. Es timates of bioburden after endoscope use range from 10^{-5} to 10^{-10} colony formin units/mL after clinical use.[13,26] Current HLD standards focus on the volumetric redu tion in bioburden using immediate post-procedure flushing and manual cleanin before automatic endoscope reprocessing (AER). However, the recent issues wi duodenoscope contamination compelled international research endeavors to op mize the current standards for reprocessing and determine whether risk mitigatic strategies may be improved.

Repeat High-Level Disinfection

Research efforts have been made to define and subsequently quantify the benefit repeating HLD as a measure of reducing contamination. Double cycle HLD cou theoretically produce a 1-log reduction of persistent contaminations based on pul lished data.[12] One high-volume endoscopy center described their protocol includir double-reprocessing with two cycles of manual cleaning and two cycles in the AE for all elevator mechanism–based scopes. EtO sterilization was reserved for ar culture-positive duodenoscopes.[27] During the study period, 329 duodenoscope were randomly selected for culture and quarantine, rather than performed per procec ure. They described a 9.1% culture rate (n = 30) with only two of those being poter tially pathogenic organisms (0.6%). A subsequent study, prospective and randomize trial of adding a second cycle of AER for all elevator mechanism–based scopes (i manual cleaning followed by single vs double cycle AER) failed to detect difference in the scope contamination rates with the added cycle.[28] These results sugges ongoing need to refine HLD practices and guidelines.

Sterilization

In 2015, the FDA suggested that health care facilities use at least one of four suc gested supplemental measures including EtO gas sterilization.[24] Some centers opte for programs aimed at complete sterilization of endoscopes, although this represen unique challenges given the heat sensitivity of endoscopes.[29] Low-temperature ste ilization methods that are currently FDA-approved include EtO gas and the liqui chemical peracetic acid.[30] AER protocols exist for EtO, glutaraldehyde, peracet acid, hydrogen peroxide, chlorine dioxide, and so forth, all of which are cumbersor because of unique, individual caveats. EtO sterilization systems have been impl mented by some endoscopy centers; however, EtO is a documented occupation hazard with carcinogenic, teratogenic, and neurotoxic effects.[31] There are also co cerning environmental impacts, as evidenced by the shutdown of a large EtO steriliz tion facility in Illinois on February 15, 2019 by the Environmental Protection Agenc because of excessive levels of the sterilant detected in ambient air sampling outsic of the facility.[32] Anecdotally, EtO sterilization has been thought to impact the functior ality of endoscopes by decreasing pliability of the scope and increasing the need fe repairs. Peracetic acid sterilization, although FDA approved, is limited by cumbersor protocols and methods that have yet to be validated for duodenoscope use.

One recent review documented that 6 of 17 outbreak sites adopted ETO sterilizatic with three sites reporting termination of the outbreak following implementation. However additional measures were taken including removing defective instrumen from service, staff remediation, scope evaluation, and repair. There are some da on the reprocessing failure rate for reprocessing sterilization, with one study reportin one positive surveillance culture for a carbapenem-resistant Enterobacteriacea

Klebsiella pneumoniae, following 592 EtO sterilization cycles.[34] The question remains whether these findings reflect a true failure of EtO sterilization rather than confirm the paramount importance of bioburden reduction during the preceding HLD.

In addition to the technical challenges of implementing a sterilization program because of logistical and environmental issues, the procedural elements require careful consideration. Residual disinfectants persisting in endoscope channels incurs the risk of potentially masking the presences of biomatter thereby obscuring accurate post-processing contamination assessments.[35] Use of a biocide neutralizer before obtaining surveillance cultures may be a necessary component of reprocessing protocols. Ex vivo studies using a narrow-lumen tubing inoculated with enteric bacteria (thereby mimicking the long working channel of a duodenoscope) demonstrated lackluster efficacy (39.7% and 35%, respectively) of gas sterilization alone without any preceding HLD.[36] Such findings support the need for stringent manual cleaning with HLD before sterilization.[37]

Biomarkers

The complexity and cumbersome nature of scope reprocessing, culturing, and/or sterilization has paved an interest in nonbiotic tissue markers, such as adenosine triphosphate, hemoglobin, and carbohydrates. These markers can be used in routine practice as a quality metric for testing reprocessing efficacy and vetting sterilization techniques. Because there are no validated processing measures, many centers have implemented such testing to assess for adequate reprocessing; however, this too may be insufficient, because adequate cleaning does not guarantee sterility.[38–40] Currently, trials using adenosine triphosphate bioluminescence have demonstrated lackluster correlation with culture results, and multiple reports of high false-negative rates using this modality limit utility as standalone surveillance method,[41] although some internal guidelines recommend consideration for use.[42]

STRATEGIES FOR RISK REDUCTION

Field users of elevator-based endoscopes remain challenged by the compulsory mission to reduce risk of infectious transmission while maintaining access to these essential procedures with fully functioning endoscopy units. Surveillance programs using serial endoscope cultures are one such strategy to detect contamination issues and early outbreaks. Adequate HLD and biofilm elimination is an efficacious method to decrease risk of infection transmission and is used as one justification for endoscope surveillance.[43] No surveillance interval or protocol has been formally validated, although many iterations of the per-procedure culture and quarantine have evolved to fit each institution's needs and resources.[44] In December 2018, the FDA published the interim analysis of the federally mandated postmarketing surveillance of duodenoscope reprocessing instructions for use from all three duodenoscope manufacturers. These initial results were notable for a higher than expected HLD defect rate of 0.4% in properly collected samples, with 3% HLD defect rate for high concern organisms. In April 2019, updated interim results were provided and reported HLD defect rates of up to 5.4% across the three scope manufacturers.[15,45] Contamination rates were even higher for improperly collected samples confirming the fallibility of such surveillance programs if performed without strict fidelity. More importantly, they suggest that despite the efforts to refine the current standard reprocessing instructions for use, the HLD defect rate remains unchanged. FDA communication updates published on August 2019 advised endoscopy centers begin transition to use of scopes with innovative designs that might reduce contamination risk or simply not require any reprocessing at all.[46] They also mandated postmarketing surveillance of the new disposable cap duodenoscopes to ensure reduction of contamination rates compared with fixed cap designs.

Despite these shortcomings, regulatory bodies including the FDA and advisory groups from Europe and Australia advise use of surveillance culturing.[42,47] There is still no consensus on optimal frequency of culturing or appropriate duration of scope quarantine when used. The Centers for Disease Control and Prevention recommends sampling after every 60 procedures if weekly or per-use culturing is not an option.[48] A standardized protocol for sampling and culturing was published in February 2018 in a joint effort by the FDA, Centers for Disease Control and Prevention, and the American Society for Microbiology; however, these protocols have yet to be validated.[48]

Beyond the technical execution of scope sampling, culture result interpretation is important for refining reprocessing measures and specific results may correspond with a lapse in scope reprocessing. A quality assurance publication from the European Society of Gastrointestinal Endoscopy (ESGE) and the European Society of Gastroenterology and Endoscopy Nurses and Associates (ESGENA) (2007) provides interpretative guidance for endoscope surveillance culture results: Enterobacteriaceae (insufficient HLD), P aeruginosa (insufficient final rinse and drying prestorage), Staphylococci sp (endoscope recontamination), Legionella sp, or atypical mycobacteria (contamination of water systems, washer-disinfector apparatus), and so forth.[42,47] It is important to remember that there remains an as yet undefined correlate between endoscope culture positivity and degree of infectivity.[49] Furthermore, endoscope reprocessing and sampling protocols are labor intensive, complicated, and therefore rife with the opportunity for human error. One method of evaluating the efficacy of HLD included assessments of germicidal activity of the glutaraldehyde component of the HLD using test strips for every five AER cycles plus scheduled servicing of the AER machinery every 3 to 6 months.[50] The numerous unvetted options leaves most centers operating without clear guidance or easily implementable strategies.

NOVEL ENDOSCOPE DESIGN
Disposable Duodenoscope Cap

In 2017 the FDA approved the Pentax Medical ED34-i10T duodenoscope featuring a sterile disposable elevator cap (DECtm), with an elevator intended for one-time, per-procedure use.[51,52] Fujifilm Corporation received FDA clearance for the duodenoscope model ED-580XT in March 2019, which also features a disposable cap.[53] The disposable cap facilitates enhanced reprocessing measures around the elevator, which has been a proven problematic area. Although advancements in device design may mitigate the contamination risk imposed by the elevator, retention of bioburden within other areas of the endoscope has proven problematic. One study using a prototype boroscope found that 23% of the endoscopes inspected postreprocessing contained intrachannel debris.[54] Nevertheless, regulatory bodies have emphasized the importance of design innovation including the recent FDA safety communication[46] from August 2019, which made formal recommendations to begin the transition away from fixed endcap duodenoscopes in favor of adopting novel scope design and technology.

Disposable Duodenoscope

The concept of a single-use duodenoscope materialized in 2018 (Exalt, single-use duodenoscope, Boston Scientific Corporation, Natick, MA) to address the multifocal contamination risk of the duodenoscope.[55] A comparative bench-simulation study nd the first human trial of the single-use instrument against three different models of eusable duodenoscopes demonstrated that in expert hands the disposable instrument performed comparably in task completion and usability.[56] The 7-day postrocedural adverse event rate for the 58 procedures was comparable with expected erious AE rate with standard duodenoscopes.[57] The implementation of one-time use echnology raises some questions given the vast application of ERCP and shear number of procedures performed annually. Additionally, the financial feasibility of stocking fully disposable instrument remains unclear. One estimation reported that the perrocedure cost of using a disposable duodenoscope at a higher volume center (perormance at the 75th percentile of ERCP volume nationally) ranged from $797 to 1547, xceeding the per-procedure cost at lower volume centers (those performing at the 5th percentile of ERCP volume nationally) with a per-procedure cost of $1318 to 068.[58] The cost analysis accounted for reusable instruments including annual procedural volume, individual scope cost and annual repair fees, scope washer and maintenance, cleaning supplies, and personnel costs all of which amounted to greater than 60,000. The study also attempted to calculate the cost of the infectious complication f cholangitis, estimated at $125,000 for hospitalizations requiring intensive care unit–evel care. The rate of infection was based on a range of rates reported as 0.4% to .0%.[1,4,12] Notably, the cost decreased significantly to $297 per scope at these higher olume centers not accounting for "infectious cost."

The ideal application for disposable endoscopes remains obscure given the disparate needs of high- versus low-volume centers, or those without adequate reprocessg facilities (ie, procedures performed on travel basis or in surgical facilities). The uestion remains if the scope use should be stratified by patient risk. Should previusly identified "high-risk patients," that is, hospitalized patients, those with cholaniocarcinoma, or biliary stent placement,[59] preferentially use the disposable istrument with the current standard instrument reserved for lower risk patient popuations? Alternatively, without embedded quality controls in the current HLD process or duodenoscopes, does risk stratification create two standards of care for patients indergoing ERCP?

UMMARY

Advancements in endoscope technology and design are needed to ensure greater afety for patients undergoing ERCP and endoscopic ultrasound. Interim solutions ave emerged to include enhanced cleaning methods, quality metrics and redundancy built into the reprocessing procedures, exhaustive informed consent, and outine maintenance of endoscopes. Such protective factors may have mitigated isk but even in combination remains an unlikely panacea. Staff training and competency must also be prioritized; however, other implementable and wholly important measures include skill task alignment, ergonomic workspace optimization, and a feedback process for all levels of staff to report system problems in a nonthreatening manner.

An obvious long-term solution is a design change eliminating the current elevator mechanism; however, even with novel designs, such as the removal duodenoscope cap or even fully disposable instruments, the feasibility of use, cost effectiveness, and long-term efficacy of these changes is yet to be determined. Another approach s to better understand how quality controls can be built into the HLD process for all endoscopes so as to identify inadequately reprocessed scopes before they reach he patient. The current standard is an imperfect tool with an imperfect method to nanage. What is clear about current scope technology is that existing endoscope manufacturer-recommended HLD protocols are inadequate to guarantee a pathogen free instrument. Optimizing current reprocessing measures, until suitable substitutions are available, remains the most judicious strategy to allow ongoing delivery of care.

Portions of the changes implemented at high-volume centers may be tailored for a smaller practice until improved duodenoscope design arises. Still needed are a validated manufacturer-recommended schedule for routine duodenoscope maintenance and reprocessing protocols that can be implemented in most endoscopy units (with reasonable equipment and operative costs). We must reconcile the risk of using an imperfect standard while impatiently awaiting the innovative evolution of these indispensable instruments.

DISCLOSURE

J.T. Higa: none. Dr A.S. Ross reports consulting fees and research funding from Boston Scientific Corporation.

REFERENCES

1. Verfaillie CJ, Bruno MJ, Voor in 't Holt AF, et al. Withdrawal of a novel-design duodenoscope ends outbreak of a VIM-2-producing *Pseudomonas aeruginosa*. Endoscopy 2015;47(6):502.
2. Wendorf KA, Kay M, Baliga C, et al. Endoscopic retrograde cholangiopancreatography-associated AmpC *Escherichia coli* outbreak. Infec Control Hosp Epidemiol 2015;36(6):634–42.
3. Smith ZL, Oh YS, Saeian K, et al. Transmission of carbapenem-resistant Enterobacteriaceae during ERCP: time to revisit the current reprocessing guidelines. Gastrointest Endosc 2015;81(4):1041–5.
4. Epstein L, Hunter JC, Arwady MA, et al. New Delhi metallo-beta-lactamase producing carbapenem-resistant *Escherichia coli* associated with exposure to duodenoscopes. JAMA 2014;312(14):1447–55.
5. Van der Bij AK, Van der Zwan D, Peirano G, et al. Metallo-beta-lactamase-producing *Pseudomonas aeruginosa* in the Netherlands: the nationwide emergence of a single sequence type. Clin Microbiol Infect 2012;18(9):E369–72.
6. Tennenbaum R, Colardelle P, Chochon M, et al. [Hepatitis C after retrograde cholangiography]. Gastroenterol Clin Biol 1993;17(10):763–4.
7. Birnie GG, Quigley EM, Clements GB, et al. Endoscopic transmission of hepatitis B virus. Gut 1983;24(2):171–4.
8. Dirlam Langlay AM, Ofstead CL, Mueller NJ, et al. Reported gastrointestinal endoscope reprocessing lapses: the tip of the iceberg. Am J Infect Control 2013;41(12):1188–94.
9. Alrabaa SF, Nguyen P, Sanderson R, et al. Early identification and control of carbapenemase-producing *Klebsiella pneumoniae*, originating from contaminated endoscopic equipment. Am J Infect Control 2013;41(6):562–4.
10. Preventable Tragedies: Superbugs and How Ineffective Monitoring of Medical Device Safety Fails Patients. United States Senate 2016; Health, Education, Labor, and Pensions Committee. Available at: https://www.help.senate.gov/imo media/doc/Duodenoscope%20Investigation%20FINAL%20Report.pdf. Accessed October 5, 2019.
11. McCool S, Clarke L, Querry A, et al. Carbapenem-resistant Enterobacteriaceae (CRE) Klebsiella pneumonia (KP) Cluster Analysis. Poster #1619. Poster presented at Infectious Disease Week/ID Week. San Francisco, CA, October 5, 2013.

12. Ross AS, Baliga C, Verma P, et al. A quarantine process for the resolution of duodenoscope-associated transmission of multidrug-resistant *Escherichia coli*. Gastrointest Endosc 2015;82(3):477–83.

13. Kovaleva J, Peters FT, van der Mei HC, et al. Transmission of infection by flexible gastrointestinal endoscopy and bronchoscopy. Clin Microbiol Rev 2013;26(2):231–54.

14. Rutala WA, Weber DJ. ERCP scopes: what can we do to prevent infections? Infect Control Hosp Epidemiol 2015;36(6):643–8.

15. United States Food and Drug Administration. The FDA provides interim results of duodenoscope reprocessing studies conducted in real-world settings: FDA Safety Communication 2018. Available at: https://www.fda.gov/medical-devices/safety-communications/fda-provides-interim-results-duodenoscope-reprocessing-studies-conducted-real-world-settings-fda. Accessed October 5, 2019.

16. Baron TH, Kozarek RA, Carr-Locke DL. ERCP. 3rd edition. Philadelphia: Elsevier; 2019.

17. Hawes R, Fockens P, Varadarajulu S. Endosonography. Chapter 2: equipment. Philadelphia: Elsevier; 2011.

18. The ECRI Society. Endoscopic retrograde cholangiopancreatography (ERCP) duodenoscopes: design may impede effective cleaning 2015. Available at: https://www.ecri.org/Resources/Superbug/CRE_Alert_022015.pdf. Accessed: September 20, 2019.

19. United States Food and Drug Administration. Factors affecting quality of reprocessing 2018. Available at: https://www.fda.gov/medical-devices/reprocessing-reusable-medical-devices/factors-affecting-quality-reprocessing. Accessed September 20, 2019.

20. Cole EC, Rutala WA, Carson JL. Evaluation of penicylinders used in disinfectant testing: bacterial attachment and surface texture. J Assoc Off Anal Chem 1987;70(5):903–6.

21. Cole EC, Rutala WA, Alfano EM. Comparison of stainless steel penicylinders used in disinfectant testing. J Assoc Off Anal Chem 1988;71(2):288–9.

22. Kovaleva J, Meessen NE, Peters FT, et al. Is bacteriologic surveillance in endoscope reprocessing stringent enough? Endoscopy 2009;41(10):913–6.

23. Pajkos A, Vickery K, Cossart Y. Is biofilm accumulation on endoscope tubing a contributor to the failure of cleaning and decontamination? J Hosp Infect 2004;58(3):224–9.

24. United States Food and Drug Administration. Supplemental measures to enhance duodenoscope reprocessing: FDASafety Communication 2015. Available at: https://www.fdanews.com/ext/resources/files/08-15/081015-duodenoscopes-fda.pdf?1520541508. Accessed September 10, 2019.

25. Asge Quality Assurance In Endoscopy Committee, Petersen BT, Chennat J, Cohen J, et al. Multisociety guideline on reprocessing flexible gastrointestinal endoscopes: 2011. Gastrointest Endosc 2011;73(6):1075–84.

26. Chu NS, Favero M. The microbial flora of the gastrointestinal tract and the cleaning of flexible endoscopes. Gastrointest Endosc Clin N Am 2000;10(2):233–44.

27. Bang JYRD, Sherman S, Webb D, et al. Impact of implementation of double-reprocessing protocol in the prevention of duodenoscope-associated carbapenem-resistant enterobacteriaceae (CRE) in a single tertiary referral center. Gastrointest Endosc 2016;83(5):AB170.

28. Bartles RL, Leggett JE, Hove S, et al. A randomized trial of single versus double high-level disinfection of duodenoscopes and linear echoendoscopes using standard automated reprocessing. Gastrointest Endosc 2018;88(2):306–13.e2.

29. Rutala WA, Weber DJ. Gastrointestinal endoscopes: a need to shift from disinfection to sterilization? JAMA 2014;312(14):1405–6.

30. Rutala WA, Weber DJ. Sterilization of endoscopic instruments: reply. JAMA 2015; 313(5):524.

31. Haney PE, Raymond BA, Lewis LC. Ethylene oxide. An occupational health hazard for hospital workers. AORN J 1990;51(2):480–1, 483, 485-486.

32. United States Environmental Protection Agency. Sterigenics Willowbrook facility - updates 2018. Available at: https://www.epa.gov/il/sterigenics-willowbrook-facility-updates. Accessed October 5, 2019.

33. Muscarella LF. Use of ethylene-oxide gas sterilisation to terminate multidrug-resistant bacterial outbreaks linked to duodenoscopes. BMJ Open Gastroenterol 2019;6(1):e000282.

34. Naryzhny I, Silas D, Chi K. Impact of ethylene oxide gas sterilization of duodenoscopes after a carbapenem-resistant Enterobacteriaceae outbreak. Gastrointest Endosc 2016;84(2):259–362.

35. Humphries RM, McDonnell G. Superbugs on duodenoscopes: the challenge of cleaning and disinfection of reusable devices. J Clin Microbiol 2015;53(10): 3118–25.

36. Alfa MJ, DeGagne P, Olson N, et al. Comparison of ion plasma, vaporized hydrogen peroxide, and 100% ethylene oxide sterilizers to the 12/88 ethylene oxide gas sterilizer. Infect Control Hosp Epidemiol 1996;17(2):92–100.

37. Rutala WA, Weber DJ. Outbreaks of carbapenem-resistant Enterobacteriaceae infections associated with duodenoscopes: what can we do to prevent infections? Am J Infect Control 2016;44(5 Suppl):e47–51.

38. Alfa MJ, Fatima I, Olson N. The adenosine triphosphate test is a rapid and reliable audit tool to assess manual cleaning adequacy of flexible endoscope channels. Am J Infect Control 2013;41(3):249–53.

39. Cloutman-Green E, Canales M, Zhou Q, et al. Biochemical and microbial contamination of surgical devices: a quantitative analysis. Am J Infect Control 2015; 43(6):659–61.

40. Hansen D, Benner D, Hilgenhoner M, et al. ATP measurement as method to monitor the quality of reprocessing flexible endoscopes. Ger Med Sci 2004;2: Doc04.

41. United States Centers for Disease Control and Prevention. Interim protocol for healthcare facilities regarding surveillance for bacterial contamination of duodenoscopes after reprocessing. CDC; 2015. Available at: http://www.cdc.gov/hai/organisms/cre/cre-duodenoscope-surveillance-protocol.html. Accessed September 20, 2019.

42. Beilenhoff U, Neumann CS, Rey JF, et al. ESGE-ESGENA guideline for quality assurance in reprocessing: microbiological surveillance testing in endoscopy. Endoscopy 2007;39(2):175–81.

43. Aumeran C, Thibert E, Chapelle FA, et al. Assessment on experimental bacterial biofilms and in clinical practice of the efficacy of sampling solutions for microbiological testing of endoscopes. J Clin Microbiol 2012;50(3):938–42.

44. Rutala WA, Weber DJ. Reprocessing semicritical items: current issues and new technologies. Am J Infect Control 2016;44(5 Suppl):e53–62.

45. United States Food and Drug Administration. Statement from Jeff Shuren, M.D., Director of the Center for Devices and Radiological Health, on continued efforts to assess duodenoscope contamination risk. 2019. Available at: https://www.fda.gov/news-events/press-announcements/statement-jeff-shuren-md-director-center-devices-and-radiological-health-continued-efforts-assess. Accessed September 5, 2019.

6. United States Food and Drug Administration. The FDA is recommending transition to duodenoscopes with innovative designs to enhance safety: FDA safety communication 2019. Available at: https://www.fda.gov/medical-devices/safety-communications/fda-recommending-transition-duodenoscopes-innovative-designs-enhance-safety-fda-safety-communication. Accessed September 5, 2019.

7. Shin SP, Kim WH. Recent update on microbiological monitoring of gastrointestinal endoscopes after high-level disinfection. Clin Endosc 2015;48(5):369–73.

8. United States Centers for Disease Control and Prevention. Duodenoscope surveillance sampling & culturing reducing the risks of infection 2015. Available at: https://www.cdc.gov/hai/organisms/cre/cre-duodenoscope-surveillance-protocol.html. Accessed September 5, 2019.

9. Gazdik MA, Coombs J, Burke JP, et al. Comparison of two culture methods for use in assessing microbial contamination of duodenoscopes. J Clin Microbiol 2016;54(2):312–6.

10. Chiu KW, Lu LS, Chiou SS. High-level disinfection of gastrointestinal endoscope reprocessing. World J Exp Med 2015;5(1):33–9.

11. Pentax Medical Announcement. Pentax medical announces launch of first FDA-cleared HD duodenoscope with disposable distal cap 2017. Available at: https://www.pentaxmedical.com/pentax/en/99/1/PENTAX-MEDICAL-ANNOUNCES-LAUNCH-OF-FIRST-FDA-CLEARED-HD-DUODENOSCOPE-WITH-DISPOSABLE-DISTAL-CAP. Accessed September 5, 2019.

12. Voelker R. Duodenoscope design aimed at infection prevention. JAMA 2017; 318(17):1644.

13. United States Food and Drug Administration. FUJIFILM duodenoscope model ED-580XT 2019. Available at: https://www.accessdata.fda.gov/cdrh_docs/pdf18/K181745.pdf. Accessed September 5, 2019.

14. Thaker AM, Kim S, Sedarat A, et al. Inspection of endoscope instrument channels after reprocessing using a prototype borescope. Gastrointest Endosc 2018; 88(4):612–9.

15. United States National Library of Medicine. Initial case series with exalt single-use duodenoscope 2018. Available at: https://clinicaltrials.gov/ct2/show/NCT03701958. Accessed September 5, 2019.

16. Ross AS, Bruno MJ, Kozarek RA, et al. A novel single-use duodenoscope performs similarly to 3 models of reusable duodenoscopes for endoscopic retrograde cholangiopancreatography: a randomized bench-model comparison. Gastrointest Endosc 2020;91(2):396–403.

17. Muthusamy VR, Bruno MJ, Kozarek RA, et al. Clinical evaluation of a single-use duodenoscope for endoscopic retrograde cholangiopancreatography. Clin Gastroenterol Hepatol 2019. https://doi.org/10.1016/j.cgh.2019.10.052.

18. Bang JY, Sutton B, Hawes R, et al. Concept of disposable duodenoscope: at what cost? Gut 2019;68(11):1915–7.

19. Kim S, Russell D, Mohamadnejad M, et al. Risk factors associated with the transmission of carbapenem-resistant Enterobacteriaceae via contaminated duodenoscopes. Gastrointest Endosc 2016;83(6):1121–9.

Methods for Endoscope Reprocessing

Neil B. Marya, MD, Raman V. Muthusamy, MD, MAS*

KEYWORDS

- Endoscope reprocessing • Automated endoscope reprocessors • Manual cleaning
- High-level disinfection • Duodenoscope

KEY POINTS

- Point-of-use precleaning, manual cleaning, leak testing, high-level disinfection, and drying/storage are the key steps of endoscope reprocessing.
- Enhancements of these various steps are being pursued to prevent endoscopic transmission of pathogenic organisms between patients.
- Although simplification and automation of the steps in the endoscope reprocessing cycle may help remove human error from the process, auditing and improving staff adherence to current reprocessing protocols is vital.

INTRODUCTION

The management of many gastrointestinal diseases relies on diagnostic and therapeutic capabilities afforded by endoscopy. On average, there are approximately 7 million upper, 12 million lower, and 700,000 biliary endoscopies performed annually in the United States.[1,2] Although endoscopic procedures carry a very minimal risk of infection, the potential transmission of exogenous infections among patients has emerged as a significant concern for patients, clinicians, health care facilities, endoscope manufacturers, and regulatory agencies.

Since 2002, more than 40 outbreaks of multidrug-resistant organisms (MDROs) attributed to endoscopic transmission have been reported by centers around the world.[3] These occurrences have primarily involved duodenoscopes and have brought to light new concerns regarding limitations in endoscope reprocessing that may be responsible for transmission of infections between patients. In some of these cases, centers reported problems with cleaning and maintenance of endoscopes and were able to create or adapt detailed protocols to stem outbreaks once the issues were identified. In many cases, however, either the detail of reporting on individual occurrences was too limited to identify causative factors or no clear breach in the established protocol was ever identified.[4-6]

Vatche and Tamar Manoukian Division of Digestive Diseases, David Geffen School of Medicine at UCLA, 200 UCLA Medical Plaza, Suite 214, Los Angeles, CA 90095, USA
* Corresponding author.
E-mail address: raman@mednet.ucla.edu

Gastrointest Endoscopy Clin N Am 30 (2020) 665–675
https://doi.org/10.1016/j.giec.2020.06.002
1052-5157/20/© 2020 Elsevier Inc. All rights reserved.

giendo.theclinics.com

The reports of these outbreaks have led to a revived focus on optimizing endoscope reprocessing. In 2016, numerous societies endorsed a revised multisociety document regarding endoscope reprocessing.[7] In their statement, the societies provided recommendations with goals to standardize endoscope reprocessing and to minimize the risk of transmitting infections between patients. The societies recommended that all centers include point-of-use precleaning, leak testing, manual cleaning, high-level disinfection (HLD), storage, and drying as part of the reprocessing cycle. However, given that several outbreaks of MDROs have occurred despite apparent adherence to recommended reprocessing cycles, concerns remain that current reprocessing techniques may not be sufficient to completely eliminate the potential risk of transmission of infections between patients.

This article will discuss the various steps and methods in the recommended HLD reprocessing cycle, as well as possible enhancements to the process that are on the horizon (**Fig. 1**). It should be noted that the steps described in this article are general guidelines and that specific reprocessing steps for endoscopes should be performed as directed in the original endoscope manufacturer (OEM) reprocessing instructions.

ENDOSCOPE CLEANING

Initial precleaning and manual cleaning are likely the most crucial aspects of successful endoscope reprocessing. The removal of organic material from the many surfaces and channels of the endoscope is essential to allowing disinfectant direct contact with underlying organisms. HLD is defined as a 6-log reduction in bacterial burden. Studies have shown that, on their own, the precleaning and manual cleaning of the endoscope can decrease bioburden by 3 to 4 logs, thus emphasizing the roles of these steps.[8] If this part of endoscope reprocessing is not given adequate attention and/or not

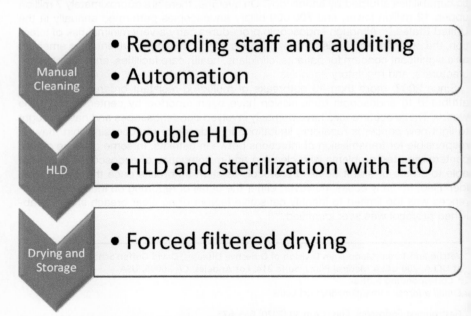

Manual Cleaning
- Recording staff and auditing
- Automation

HLD
- Double HLD
- HLD and sterilization with EtO

Drying and Storage
- Forced filtered drying

Fig. 1. Endoscope reprocessing cycle with potential enhancements for each step that have been studied. EtO, ethylene oxide; HLD, high-level disinfection.

erformed correctly, whatever occurs thereafter during the remainder of the cleaning ycle can be rendered moot no matter the length of disinfectant exposure time. As discussed in this section, a major focus of quality improvement efforts is to improve eprocessing focus on the precleaning and manual cleaning steps. Technicians and urses responsible for cleaning must therefore undergo dedicated training and competency verification to ensure that proper scope cleaning is performed as recommended by current guidelines and OEM instructions.

recleaning

Before cleaning, staff should make sure they are wearing adequate protective gear because the various detergents and chemicals used for manual cleaning can be severe irritants to skin and mucous membranes. Those involved in manual cleaning should be required to wear gowns and gloves and should also ideally wear protective eyewear or face shields.

Immediately following the completion of the endoscopic procedure (although the ndoscope is still connected to the processor), staff should wipe the scope with a loth immersed in an enzymatic solution. Next, a detergent (separate from the previously mentioned enzymatic solution) should be flushed through both the air/water channel and the instrument channel of the scope. If a dual-channel scope is being cleaned, then both instrument channels must be suctioned and cleaned regardless f whether the channel was instrumented during the procedure. Finally, all detachable parts of the endoscope must be removed (ie, the biopsy port and air/water and suction alves).

Individual endoscopy units may choose to either purchase disposable, single-use valves and ports or use reusable parts. Endoscopy staff must be familiar with the specific practice and device accessories that are being used in their department. If a part s meant to be single-use, it should be disposed of once precleaning is complete. If, however, the valves and ports are reusable, they should instead be immersed in the enzymatic detergent with further reprocessing performed as indicated by the part manufacturer.[9] Once the precleaning is complete, the endoscope can then be taken rom the procedure room to the designated reprocessing area.

Staff should also be instructed that reprocessing should begin as soon as the procedure is completed so that the bioburden on the scope is not given time to harden, making removal more difficult. If there is an emergency case performed overnight, it may not be possible for reprocessing to be performed immediately depending on the resources available at an institution. In such situations, at an absolute minimum, precleaning (as described earlier) should be performed and the endoscope should soak in the enzymatic detergent until full reprocessing can be performed at a later time.

Staff should be aware, however, that extended soaks should be infrequent and kept as short as possible and should not in any circumstance exceed 10 hours. Prolonged soaks carry a risk of permitting bioburden to set, allowing biofilm to form. Furthermore, this practice is potentially damaging to the structural integrity of the endoscope and may cause leaks. It is therefore essential that the manual cleaning process be started as soon as possible.[10]

.eak Testing

Before initiating manual cleaning, it is vital that leak testing be performed. Leak testing allows for openings in the endoscope to be identified that, over time, serve as entry points for liquids, chemicals, and organic material into the internal portions of the endoscope. Leak testing requires its own dedicated training for staff and can be a source of human error. At least one outbreak of *Mycobacterium tuberculosis* has been attributed to a failure of staff to detect a leak that was later identified by the scope manufacturer.[11] Endoscope staff should be aware that although larger leaks may be obvious to the naked eye, smaller leaks require more dutiful examination. The most common leak tests performed include a dry leak test and a manual wet leak test.

The first step of any leak test is to make sure that water caps are placed over the electrical contacts of the scopes. This helps prevent these components from being damaged and helps eliminate fluid invasion. During a dry leak test, a manual or automatic leak tester is attached to the scope channels. Positive air pressure is then introduced into the scope to assess scope integrity. When using a manual tester, staff are instructed to assess an attached barometer for signs of pressure loss, which indicates a scope leak.

During a wet leak test, the internal channels of the endoscope are flushed with water and the external surface of the endoscope is irrigated with water to remove any bubbles. Once this is complete, the bending section and then the entire scope is submerged in water. Next, although the scope is underwater, the internal channels are flushed with water. Over the course of the next several minutes, staff should be closely observing for bubbles indicating the presence of a scope leak.[12]

In addition to leak testing, it is further recommended that staff closely inspect the distal tip of the endoscope to look for any defects. The importance of this step has been highlighted by reports of contaminated endoscopes that had passed the leak test, but through close inspection of the distal tip by the scope manufacturer they were found to have defects.[5,13,14] These reports underscore that leak testing alone is not sufficient to rule out scope defects that can result in cross-contamination.

Manual Cleaning

Once leak testing is complete, the scope should be kept in the decontamination room and manual cleaning performed. To start, a fresh detergent is poured into a clean basin in which the endoscope is eventually submerged. All debris is removed from the external surface of the endoscope using brushes and wipes. Soft, small brushes are used to clean all removable parts. Brushes are then used to clean the channels of the endoscope. Care must be taken to use brush sizes compatible with channels as recommended by the scope manufacturer. Adapters are then connected to the suction and air/water channels of the scope allowing for the detergent solution to be flushed through. Staff should be aware that some scopes require additional adapters. Duodenoscopes, for example, require an adapter specific for the elevator channel. The scope should then be immersed in the detergent solution for a period of time as specified by the product label.

Once all of these steps are complete, the scope should be irrigated with sterile water to remove any residual debris or cleaning solution. Water should then be removed from the channels with forced air and the external surface dried with wipes and cloths.

Future Directions in Pre-High-Level Disinfection Cleaning

The initial cleaning aspects of endoscope reprocessing have been a focus of much research and quality improvement efforts. Although some researchers have suggested moving completely to automation and removing any manual cleaning steps from the reprocessing cycle,[15] the effectiveness of automated cleaning has yet to be adequately determined. For example, one study comparing automated versus manual cleaning of laparoscopic instruments failed to show any difference in detectable organic residues between the 2 modalities.[16] Although we await further study into the potential role of automated cleaners of endoscopes, centers can focus on how to improve manual cleaning of endoscopes by aiming to minimize the potential for human error. One study by Armellino and colleagues investigated the impact of video monitoring and auditing of staff members during the manual cleaning process. In this study, auditors were shown a live video feed of staff members cleaning duodenoscopes and scored staff using a 15-point check list. During the first week of assessment, staff members were found to achieve a compliance rate of only 53.1% for all reprocessing steps. Once staff received feedback and reeducation based on the findings from the auditors, compliance rates increased to 98.9%.[17] Further studies are needed to assess common deficiencies in manual cleaning and to better understand what modalities are most effective in optimizing staff adherence to cleaning protocols. Clarifying the instructions for reprocessing the devices and simplification of the steps involved in manual cleaning would likely also be beneficial in improving this process.

HIGH-LEVEL DISINFECTION

Based on the Spaulding classification, devices used in gastrointestinal endoscopy are considered "semicritical" and therefore require HLD.[7,18] Traditionally, HLD is defined as the eradication of all microorganisms (with the exception of some bacterial spores that may remain in cases of heavy inoculation). The Food and Drug Administration (FDA) further has defined HLD as a process by which a 6-log reduction in *Mycobacteria* species is achieved.[19] HLD involves immersing the endoscope in a chemical sterilant. Subsequently the endoscope channels are rinsed, flushed with alcohol, and then dried. HLD can be performed either manually or through automation, and different chemical cleaning solutions can be used. Given the large number of outbreaks over the past several years, experts are questioning whether current HLD practices are sufficient for reprocessing of duodenoscopes and what the optimal practice would be. In this section, the authors discuss currently used and studied HLD techniques.

Manual High-Level Disinfection and Automated Endoscope Reprocessors

As noted earlier, HLD can be performed manually or using an automated endoscope reprocessor (AER). There are many advantages to using an AER over performing HLD manually. Performing HLD manually exposes the reprocessing cycle to potential human error and also exposes staff members to potential health risks. One study by Ofstead and colleagues included a prospective analysis of the benefits of AERs compared with those of manual cleaning. The study found that personnel performing manual HLD adhered to cleaning guidelines only 1.4% of the time compared with a 75.4% adherence rate for those using AERs. The investigators also demonstrated that staff members performing manual HLD reported significantly more health issues compared with those using AER. These issues included physical injuries as well as symptoms related to inhaling the chemicals used in HLD.[20] Although there may be concern about the cost of purchasing and maintaining an AER machine, research has suggested that there is a financial benefit to using an AER over manual HLD. One study performed a financial modeling analysis and demonstrated that the savings from using an AER quickly offset the initial purchase and maintenance costs and overall had a positive financial impact compared with manual HLD.[21]

Although several companies manufacture AER models, most AERs generally function similarly. Endoscopes are submerged in a basin with the HLD cleaning solution and then connected via special hookups to the AER. This allows for the cleaning solution to be flushed through the internal channels, which are then later rinsed. Given the urgency to ensure that AER devices were capable of meeting the challenges of flexible endoscope reprocessing, the FDA requested that the 5 main manufacturers of AERs perform efficacy validation studies. For these studies, the FDA determined an AER to be successful if it was able to reduce 99.9999% of the most resistant organisms from several different parts of the duodenoscope. The FDA also recommended that AER manufacturers clearly state their methodology so that users can reproduce their level of efficacy. In following this recommendation, manufacturers often designate that hospitals use a specific HLD solution for their particular AER.

Cleaning Solutions

As indicated earlier, HLD solutions used in AERs are capable of removing all organisms (including mycobacteria, viruses, and fungi) with the exception of some bacterial spores. Various cleaning solutions available for use in HLD with AERs include glutaraldehyde, ortho-phthalaldehyde, hydrogen peroxide, and peracetic acid. Each of these solutions has advantages and disadvantages (**Table 1**), and historically, the most commonly used HLD solution has been glutaraldehyde.[22]

Glutaraldehyde has been popular because it is relatively inexpensive and causes very minimal damage to the endoscope. Limitations of glutaraldehyde include the potential for irritating the eyes and skin, along with long dwell times needed to eliminate pathogenic organisms.[23] Glutaraldehyde typically requires a 20-minute dwell time to eliminate most organisms, 45 minutes for mycobacteria, and more than 6 hours to eliminate spores. This soak time does not prohibit the use of glutaraldehyde in AERs.[24] Ortho-phthalaldehyde is another aldehyde sterilant used in AERs that avoids some of the limitations associated with glutaraldehyde. Specifically, ortho-

Table 1
Comparison of different sterilization solutions used in endoscope reprocessing

Chemical Sterilant	Time Required for Intended Effect	Pros	Cons
Glutaraldehyde	20 min to remove most organisms 6 h to eliminate spores	Inexpensive Results in minimal damage to endoscopes	Causes irritation to eyes and skin Long dwell time needed for sterilization
Ortho-phthalaldehyde	5 min	Short dwell time Not toxic	Very expensive Can permanently stain skin and clothing
Peracetic acid	10 min	Short dwell time Not toxic Inexpensive	Corrosion of metal portions of endoscopes
Ethylene Oxide	16 h	Excellent antimicrobial activity	Long sterilization process that can be challenging logistically Very toxic/known carcinogen Most hospitals require that scopes be send off-site Not available in all states May stiffen scopes Rigorous drying needed to avoid antifreeze formation

hthalaldehyde only requires an immersion time of 5 minutes and is far less toxic than lutaraldehyde.[25] Drawbacks of ortho-phthalaldehyde include its high cost and the act that it can permanently stain uncovered skin. As ortho-phthalaldehyde, peracetic cid also requires a much shorter immersion time. To eliminate most bacteria, perace-c acid only requires about 10 minutes of immersion. Unlike ortho-phthalaldehyde or lutaraldehyde, peracetic acid often is paired with another cleaning solution (such as ydrogen peroxide) to create a synergistic effect. The limitation of using peracetic acid s that its high acidity can actually corrode the metal portions of endoscopes.[26]

ouble High-Level Disinfection

s the authors continue to experiment with new ways to combat challenges with cope disinfection, one proposed change to current methods is to simply perform a econd, repeat HLD for endoscopes. For double HLD, both the manual cleaning cycle nd the HLD cycle in an AER are repeated. The possible benefits were studied in 2 ifferent randomized controlled trials performed by Snyder and colleagues and Bartles nd colleagues. In both studies, the investigators randomized elevator-containing en-loscopes to receive single HLD and double HLD. Neither study demonstrated that louble HLD resulted in any benefit in decontamination.[27,28] In another recent study, Rex and colleagues assessed the benefit of double HLD by randomly culturing the luodenoscope elevator after cleaning cycles. They found that performing double ILD alone resulted in a 0.8% rate of detection of known pathogens following elevator ulture. They also demonstrated that changing personnel along with double HLD esulted in even more improvement as the detection rate of known pathogens drop-ed further to 0.2%. The summary findings of this study indicate that although double ILD produced generally low contamination rates, it did not completely eliminate all athogens from the duodenoscope elevator channel. The study also further empha-izes that human error plays a role in scope cleaning efficacy.[29]

thylene Oxide

Ine proposed method to improve on the results of HLD and limit the possibility of hu-nan error in scope reprocessing is to perform gas sterilization with ethylene oxide EtO). Although not mandated by the FDA, several hospital systems have moved to :tO sterilization in an attempt to prevent future outbreaks. Although EtO sterilization offers excellent antimicrobial activity, as HLD, this method has a potential to incom-oletely remove bacterial spores from endoscope channels. This issue was well lemonstrated in a study by Naryzhny and colleagues. After their institution instituted EtO sterilization, duodenoscopes were randomly sampled on a monthly basis over the course of a year to assess for Carbapenem-resistant Enterobacteriaceae (CRE) contamination. During that year, they identified that one of their duodenoscopes ested positive for CRE. Following a repeat EtO sterilization, the duodenoscope even-ually tested negative.[30] In another study, EtO sterilization did not prove more effective han current commonly used methods. Snyder and colleagues randomized duodeno-scopes to receive single HLD, double HLD, as well as combined HLD/EtO sterilization. The analysis demonstrated that there was no significant improvement in decontami-nation from HLD/EtO sterilization when compared with single HLD; however, the rates of contamination by culture were high in all 3 arms and it is not clear if the organisms cultured were pathogenic or environmental, representing possible sampling error ather than true residual device contamination.[27]

In addition to concerns of whether EtO provides complete adequate sterilization of endoscopes, there are logistic issues to consider as well before adopting this method. First, if endoscopes are not sufficiently dried, the moisture within the channels can interact with EtO and produce ethylene glycol (also known as antifreeze). Next, EtO is a known carcinogen that has been associated with infertility. Its use therefore requires a facility that can carefully monitor vapor levels and handle spills in order to prevent deleterious effects on the surrounding public. Because these health concerns, state regulatory agencies are considering how to monitor facilities that perform EtO sterilization. The state of Illinois, for example, recently passed a law that bans facilities that use EtO from the state unless they can prove that all emissions from the sterilization are kept in the facility. Furthermore, these facilities must present evidence from scope manufacturers to prove that EtO sterilization is the only method available to provide adequate decontamination of the medical device.

Along with public health, EtO sterilization can also harm the scopes involved in reprocessing. In the previously cited study by Naryzhny and colleagues[30] the investigators reported that the use of EtO was associated with damage to 4 of their 6 duodenoscopes. As an additional drawback, the time required for EtO may be prohibitive for some facilities, as the sterilization process typically takes approximately 16 hours because sterilized endoscopes must be adequately ventilated before they can be used again. Thus, if a facility was to adopt sterilization by EtO, it would likely have to consider purchasing more endoscopes to ensure sufficient equipment due to the added time needed for reprocessing.

DRYING AND STORAGE

The final step of the reprocessing cycle is to store and dry the endoscopes. As discussed earlier, the efforts to optimize reprocessing studies have mostly focused on improving HLD, but few have addressed methods to improve the storing and drying of endoscopes. Studies have demonstrated that 28% to 43% of endoscopes had residual moisture after reprocessing and drying was completed.[31,32] There are concerns that residual moisture in working channels could allow for bacteria to proliferate and organize to form biofilms. Thus, some have begun studying the effect of forced air drying on residual moisture in endoscopes.

Forced Filtered Air-drying Cabinets

The authors recently reported on the effect of a forced filtered air cabinet on decreasing bacterial contamination for different flexible endoscopes over time. In this study the authors demonstrated that internal working channels for endoscopes stored in standard cabinets were dry after 24 hours, whereas those connected to a forced filtered air cabinet were dry in 1 hour. The study also showed that the external surface of endoscopes took more than 24 hours to dry in standard cabinets, but those in the forced filtered air cabinet were dry in 3 hours. Finally, it was also found that forced filtered air cabinets significantly reduce bacterial proliferation in presoiled devices when compared with standard cabinets.[33]

SUMMARY

In this article, the authors have reviewed the basics of endoscope reprocessing while also addressing recent research efforts that have been undertaken to improve standard practices. One commonality that links many of these research projects is a focus on automation and removing the possibility of human error from the reprocessing cycle. Although there is clear evidence that the potential for human error is present during the manual cleaning phase, the HLD phase, and the drying phase, there is also evidence that video evaluation and subsequent reeducation of staff can have a major positive impact on successful reprocessing. Thus, although it is important to consider new technologies and chemicals that could augment reprocessing, it must not be forgetten that properly training staff members is of great value. A final message to take away from this article is that research must be focused on improving all steps of the reprocessing cycle. Simply changing a chemical or an AER is likely to be insufficient. If we are to truly achieve our goal to zero infections transmitted among patients via endoscopes, we must approach redesigning the reprocessing cycle from all possible angles.

DISCLOSURE

Dr N.B. Marya is a consultant for AnX Robotica. Dr V.R. Muthusamy is a consultant for Boston Scientific, Medivators, Interpace and Medtronic; honoraria recipient from Torax Medical and receives research support from Boston Scientific and Medtronic.

REFERENCES

1. Peery AF, Dellon ES, Lund J, et al. Burden of gastrointestinal disease in the United States: 2012 update. Gastroenterology 2012;143:1179–1187 e3.
2. Cote GA, Singh S, Bucksot LG, et al. Association between volume of endoscopic retrograde cholangiopancreatography at an academic medical center and use of pancreatobiliary therapy. Clin Gastroenterol Hepatol 2012;10:920–4.
3. Rubin ZA, Kim S, Thaker AM, et al. Safely reprocessing duodenoscopes: current evidence and future directions. Lancet Gastroenterol Hepatol 2018;3:499–508.
4. Robertson P, Smith A, Anderson M, et al. Transmission of Salmonella enteritidis after endoscopic retrograde cholangiopancreatography because of inadequate endoscope decontamination. Am J Infect Control 2017;45:440–2.
5. Epstein L, Hunter JC, Arwady MA, et al. New Delhi metallo-beta-lactamase-producing carbapenem-resistant Escherichia coli associated with exposure to duodenoscopes. JAMA 2014;312:1447–55.
6. Alrabaa SF, Nguyen P, Sanderson R, et al. Early identification and control of carbapenemase-producing Klebsiella pneumoniae, originating from contaminated endoscopic equipment. Am J Infect Control 2013;41:562–4.
7. Petersen BT, Cohen J, Hambrick RD III, et al. Multisociety guideline on reprocessing flexible GI endoscopes: 2016 update. Gastrointest Endosc 2017;85: 282–94.e1.
8. Martiny H, Floss H, Zuhlsdorf B. The importance of cleaning for the overall results of processing endoscopes. J Hosp Infect 2004;56(Suppl 2):S16–22.
9. Society of Gastroenterology N, Associates. Reprocessing of endoscopic accessories and valves. Gastroenterol Nurs 2013;36:291–2.
10. Alfa MJ, Howie R. Modeling microbial survival in buildup biofilm for complex medical devices. BMC Infect Dis 2009;9:56.
11. Ramsey AH, Oemig TV, Davis JP, et al. An outbreak of bronchoscopy-related Mycobacterium tuberculosis infections due to lack of bronchoscope leak testing. Chest 2002;121:976–81.
12. Beilenhoff U, Biering H, Blum R, et al. Prevention of multidrug-resistant infections from contaminated duodenoscopes: Position Statement of the European Society of Gastrointestinal Endoscopy (ESGE) and European Society of Gastroenterology Nurses and Associates (ESGENA). Endoscopy 2017;49:1098–106.
13. Kola A, Piening B, Pape UF, et al. An outbreak of carbapenem-resistant OXA-48 - producing Klebsiella pneumonia associated to duodenoscopy. Antimicrob Resist Infect Control 2015;4:8.

14. Verfaillie CJ, Bruno MJ, Voor in 't Holt AF, et al. Withdrawal of a novel-design duodenoscope ends outbreak of a VIM-2-producing Pseudomonas aeruginosa. Endoscopy 2015;47:493–502.

15. Ofstead CL, Wetzler HP, Doyle EM, et al. Persistent contamination on colonoscopes and gastroscopes detected by biologic cultures and rapid indicators despite reprocessing performed in accordance with guidelines. Am J Infect Control 2015;43:794–801.

16. de Camargo TC, Almeida A, Bruna CQM, et al. Manual and automated cleaning are equally effective for the removal of organic contaminants from laparoscopic instruments. Infect Control Hosp Epidemiol 2018;39:58–63.

17. Armellino D, Cifu K, Wallace M, et al. Implementation of remote video auditing with feedback and compliance for manual-cleaning protocols of endoscopic retrograde cholangiopancreatography endoscopes. Am J Infect Control 2018; 46:594–6.

18. Spaulding EH. Chemical disinfection of medical and surgical materials. Philadelphia: Lea & Febiger; 1968.

19. Committee AT, Parsi MA, Sullivan SA, et al. Automated endoscope reprocessors. Gastrointest Endosc 2016;84:885–92.

20. Ofstead CL, Wetzler HP, Snyder AK, et al. Endoscope reprocessing methods: a prospective study on the impact of human factors and automation. Gastroenterol Nurs 2010;33:304–11.

21. Funk SE, Reaven NL. High-level endoscope disinfection processes in emerging economies: financial impact of manual process versus automated endoscope reprocessing. J Hosp Infect 2014;86:250–4.

22. Society of Gastroenterology N, Associates. SGNA guidelines for nursing care of the patient receiving sedation and analgesia in the gastrointestinal endoscopy setting. Gastroenterol Nurs 2000;23:125–9.

23. Cowan RE, Manning AP, Ayliffe GA, et al. Aldehyde disinfectants and health in endoscopy units. British Society of Gastroenterology Endoscopy Committee. Gut 1993;34:1641–5.

24. Griffiths PA, Babb JR, Fraise AP. Mycobactericidal activity of selected disinfectants using a quantitative suspension test. J Hosp Infect 1999;41:111–21.

25. Alfa MJ, Sitter DL. In-hospital evaluation of orthophthalaldehyde as a high level disinfectant for flexible endoscopes. J Hosp Infect 1994;26:15–26.

26. Park S, Jang JY, Koo JS, et al. A review of current disinfectants for gastrointestinal endoscopic reprocessing. Clin Endosc 2013;46:337–41.

27. Snyder GM, Wright SB, Smithey A, et al. Randomized comparison of 3 high-level disinfection and sterilization procedures for duodenoscopes. Gastroenterology 2017;153:1018–25.

28. Bartles RL, Leggett JE, Hove S, et al. A randomized trial of single versus double high-level disinfection of duodenoscopes and linear echoendoscopes using standard automated reprocessing. Gastrointest Endosc 2018;88:306–13.e2.

29. Rex DK, Sieber M, Lehman GA, et al. A double-reprocessing high-level disinfection protocol does not eliminate positive cultures from the elevators of duodenoscopes. Endoscopy 2017;50(6):588–96.

30. Naryzhny I, Silas D, Chi K. Impact of ethylene oxide gas sterilization of duodenoscopes after a carbapenem-resistant Enterobacteriaceae outbreak. Gastrointest Endosc 2016;84:259–62.

31. Barakat MT, Girotra M, Huang RJ, et al. Scoping the scope: endoscopic evaluation of endoscope working channels with a new high-resolution inspection endoscope (with video). Gastrointest Endosc 2018;88:601–611 e1.

2. Thaker AM, Kim S, Sedarat A, et al. Inspection of endoscope instrument channels after reprocessing using a prototype borescope. Gastrointest Endosc 2018; 88(4):612–9.

3. Perumpail RB, Marya NB, McGinty BL, et al. Endoscope reprocessing: Comparison of drying effectiveness and microbial levels with an automated drying and storage cabinet with forced filtered air and a standard storage cabinet. Am J Infect Control 2019;47(9):1083–9.

Novel Algorithms for Reprocessing, Drying and Storing Endoscopes

Monique T. Barakat, MD, PhD, Subhas Banerjee, MD*

KEYWORDS

- Endoscope reprocessing • Endoscope transmitted infections • Endoscope drying
- Endoscope storage

KEY POINTS

- There is increasing recognition that standard endoscope reprocessing practices may not represent the ideal approach for preventing endoscope-transmitted infections.
- The optimal enhanced duodenoscope reprocessing modality remains to be determined and is an area in need of further research.
- Duodenoscopes with innovative designs that allow more effective reprocessing, such as duodenoscopes with detachable disposable endcaps or entirely disposable distal tips, which include the elevator address many of the limitations to effective duodenoscope reprocessing.
- In the absence of definitive data, and while anticipating the eventual availability of additional data and guidelines, each institution must decide which approach(es) to surveillance and enhanced duodenoscope reprocessing are most appropriate locally, based on the procedure volume, the background MDRO infection rates at the institution and on institutional budgetary constraints.

The Spaulding system classifies medical devices as noncritical, semicritical, or critical based on the risk of transmission of infection related to their use,[1] which in turn determines the level of reprocessing necessary after their use. Noncritical devices only make contact with skin (eg, oximeter, blood pressure cuffs) and standard cleaning is considered adequate for these devices. Critical devices enter sterile tissue or vascular spaces (eg, biopsy forceps, biopsy needles). Such devices should be sterilized or be disposed after a single use. Semicritical devices make contact with mucous

Division of Gastroenterology and Hepatology, Stanford University School of Medicine, Stanford, CA 94305, USA
* Corresponding author. Division of Gastroenterology and Hepatology, Stanford University School of Medicine, 300 Pasteur Drive, MC 5244, Stanford, CA 94305.
E-mail address: sbanerje@stanford.edu

Gastrointest Endoscopy Clin N Am 30 (2020) 677–691
https://doi.org/10.1016/j.giec.2020.06.003
giendo.theclinics.com
1052-5157/20/© 2020 Elsevier Inc. All rights reserved.

membranes (eg, gastrointestinal endoscopes). These devices require high-level disinfection (HLD) for reprocessing.

The classification of flexible endoscopes as semicritical devices has been fortuitous because, given their material composition and design, endoscopes are not temperature resistant and cannot undergo the high temperature steam sterilization processes typically used for surgical instruments.[2] This prevailing status quo is now facing challenges. Over the past few years, duodenoscopes have been associated with outbreaks of infection and some experts have called for their reclassification as critical devices, given that these endoscopes and associated devices commonly contact nonintact mucous membranes and sterile tissue.[3]

REPROCESSING OF ENDOSCOPES

Endoscope reprocessing is a complex, multistage process, with broad steps including point-of-use precleaning, manual cleaning, and HLD followed by alcohol flushing and drying.[2]

Standard Reprocessing

Point-of-use precleaning
This step is performed in the endoscopy room immediately after completion of the procedure and includes washing the external surface of the endoscope with enzymatic detergent solution and suctioning this solution through the biopsy/suction channel. The air/water channel is then purged to clear debris from the channel. This is an important foundational step in adequate endoscope reprocessing in that it decreases the initial bacterial burden within the endoscope significantly and prevents debris and tissue from drying on the outer surface of the endoscope and within the endoscope channels.[4]

Manual cleaning
Manual cleaning is performed by immersing the endoscope in fresh detergent solution while debris is removed from the external surface and from all channels using wipes/brushes.[2] For endoscopes with elevators (duodenoscopes and linear echoendoscopes), the elevator mechanism at the distal tip of the endoscope must be cleaned thoroughly and be free of any debris when examined with elevator in both the open/up and closed/down positions. To conduct leak testing, the internal endoscope channels are filled with air and the endoscope is submerged in water and observed for any bubbles emanating from the external surface or channel ports. If any leak is evident, the endoscope is sent to the manufacturer for additional testing and repair. The endoscope is then rinsed with clean water to remove debris and detergent.

High-level disinfection
HLD is performed manually, or increasingly, by use of an automated endoscope reprocessor (AER), which is programmed to circulate liquid chemical germicides (eg, glutaraldehyde, peracetic acid, hydrogen peroxide, orthophthaldehyde), alternating with alcohol and sterile water through the endoscope channels and over the external surface of the endoscope. HLD must be performed with strict adherence to endoscope manufacturer recommendations. Some of the AER solutions are reused, with testing for potency of the solutions between reprocessing cycles.

Water/alcohol flushes and drying are performed after HLD. The external surface of the endoscope is washed and the internal endoscope channels are flushed with sterile water, then with isopropyl alcohol (70%–80%). Forced air drying of the external

urface of the endoscope, followed by contact drying with a lint-free towel is then undertaken and filtered air is then flushed through endoscope working channels using air
guns or automated drying devices.[5]

These extensive endoscope reprocessing efforts are expensive and time
consuming, with the average estimated hands-on time required to reprocess a single
endoscope estimated at 76 minutes.[6] The estimated overall cost of reprocessing a
single flexible endoscope has ranged from $114.07 to $280.71.[6]

MONITORING THE EFFICACY OF ENDOSCOPE REPROCESSING
Adenosine Triphosphate Bioluminescence Testing

Adenosine triphosphate (ATP) is present in micro-organisms as well as in human cells,
and its detection offers a rapid and easy method to detect microbial/biological residue
in endoscopes. Results from ATP testing are available within a few minutes and the
process of ATP testing and interpretation does not require significant additional
training or expertise. Several commercial systems for ATP testing are available at relatively low cost.[5] ATP testing has been validated for endoscope surveillance after
manual cleaning, and before HLD.[7–9] However, it would be optimal to have a testing
mechanism for endoscopes to ensure they have low bioburden levels immediately
before patient use. This factor has prompted study of the usefulness of ATP testing
after HLD. Several groups have now studied and described ATP bioluminescence
for endoscope surveillance after HLD.[10–15]

Although ATP testing can be performed conveniently, rapidly, and at low cost, it has
some noteworthy limitations. Although low ATP bioluminescence values are reassuring, they do not unequivocally indicate that endoscope working channels are free of
microbial residue.[16,17] Conventional microbial culture seems to be more sensitive
than ATP bioluminescence. Moreover, a recent US Food and Drug Administration
(FDA) safety communication advised that ATP test strips should not be used to assess
duodenoscope cleaning, given that the FDA has not yet evaluated them for effectiveness for assessing duodenoscope reprocessing.[18] The FDA, however, urged manufacturers of ATP test strips to submit data to support the marketing of these strips
for this use.

Bioburden assays

In addition to ATP bioluminescence assays, other assays are available for rapid evaluation for residual bioburden within endoscope working channels. These modalities
(Scope-Check, Valisafe America, Tampa, FL; EndoCheck, and ChannelCheck,
HealthMark Industries, Fraser, MI) test for residue on endoscope surfaces and within
endoscope working channels. Scope-Check is an assay for protein residue on endoscope surfaces, EndoCheck detects protein and blood residue within the endoscope
working channel and ChannelCheck detects protein, blood and carbohydrate residue
within the endoscope working channel. These test strips hold potential for assessment
of the adequacy of manual cleaning before HLD. Similar to ATP bioluminescence
testing, these tests are easily performed and the assays are rapid, with results available within minutes.[5] Benchmarks for organic bioburden residue detection after
manual cleaning and before HLD have been established.[19] A simulated use study evaluating a prototype rapid use scope test strip to determine the efficacy of manual
cleaning for flexible endoscope channels, validated the ability of this test strip to
detect levels of bioburden residue above these thresholds, reflective of improperly
cleaned endoscopes.[19] This modality was then tested in the clinical setting, with 44
endoscopy centers using the test strip and 1489 endoscope channels tested;

96.6% were negative, which was interpreted to indicate that the proposed benchmark thresholds were appropriate.[19]

Endoscope cultures

As a measure of adequacy of endoscope reprocessing and to prevent transmission of infection, culture protocols have been developed and implemented at some institutions. Nevertheless, endoscope cultures for microbial surveillance have been controversial and potentially prone to environmental contamination.[14] Routine microbial surveillance is recommended by the European Society of Gastrointestinal Endoscopy and the Gastroenterological Society of Australia.[20,21] Surveillance culture protocols were not initially endorsed by the 2016 multisociety guidelines for endoscope reprocessing.[4] As a step toward valid and uniform approaches to microbial surveillance of endoscopes, the FDA and the American Society of Microbiology subsequently partnered to develop duodenoscope surveillance sampling and culturing protocols in 2018.[22]

The surveillance culture approach involves testing endoscopes in use within the endoscopy unit on an intermittent basis to determine an estimate of the rate of culture positivity. Each endoscope may be cultured once or twice per month in accordance with this protocol. Endoscopes from which cultures have been obtained are often quarantined while culture results are pending, but this step would be expected to have minimal impact on endoscopy workflow in a unit, given the small number of endoscopes undergoing culture and quarantine simultaneously, if any, within the unit.

BARRIERS TO ADEQUATE REPROCESSING

Human Factors

Human error is perhaps the most common element of deficiencies in endoscope reprocessing. Human lapses in the manual steps of endoscope reprocessing may contribute to endoscopy-associated infections.[23] Targeted training has been shown to improve adherence to best practices for manual steps of endoscope cleaning.[11] A 2010 multisite observational report indicated only 1.4% complete adherence to all steps and details of endoscope reprocessing guidelines when endoscopes were reprocessed using manual cleaning methods, in comparison with a 75.4% adherence to guidelines when an AER was used.[23] Thus, standardization and automation of processes will minimize the impact of human lapses. Based on this principle, the Centers for Disease Control and Prevention issued a statement endorsing the benefits of automated endoscope reprocessing over manual HLD.[24] However, even when an AER is used for HLD, the crucially important manual cleaning steps preceding HLD and drying steps after HLD will remain susceptible to human lapses. Efforts to minimize manual steps in endoscope reprocessing could potentially minimize the risk of endoscope-associated transmission of infection.

Simethicone Use

Simethicone is insoluble in both water and alcohol, yet is ubiquitously used for clearance of bubbles to enhance visualization during endoscopy.[25] Two separate groups have demonstrated that simethicone injected into the endoscope working channel during endoscopy is retained in these working channels after reprocessing.[25,26] An institution where simethicone was routinely added to the irrigation water bottle reported finding of simethicone-associated crystals within the waterjet channels of all colonoscopes in use.[27] Irrigation with higher concentrations of simethicone through endoscope working channels is associated with a higher number of retained fluid droplets and higher ATP bioluminescence values within these channels after reprocessing and drying, compared with when lower concentrations of simethicone or water are used.[25] However simethicone remains detectable in endoscope working channels after reprocessing, even when low concentrations are used.[25] The association between use of higher concentrations of simethicone and increased fluid and bioburden retention within endoscope working channels despite standard endoscope reprocessing underscores the importance of limiting the use of simethicone and, when necessary, using the minimum concentration necessary. Two cycles of endoscope reprocessing after the use of medium- or high-concentration simethicone resulted in a lower number of retained fluid droplets and ATP bioluminescence within endoscope working channels, when compared with endoscopes that had undergone a single cycle of reprocessing.[25]

Undetected Internal Damage of Endoscopes

Recent outbreaks of duodenoscope-related infection suggest that it may be difficult to detect small foci of endoscope damage particularly within internal channels.[28–32] A recent study conducted at a high-volume endoscopic retrograde cholangiopancreatography medical center reported that the withdrawal of specific duodenoscopes with a high rate of culture positivity contributed to an overall decrease in the HLD defect rate at their institution.[8] The inability to achieve adequate HLD despite repeated cycles of reprocessing in some duodenoscopes may relate to damage within their internal channels. Such areas of damage may be difficult to adequately clean and disinfect and may serve as a sanctuary for bacterial proliferation.

Inspection of the duodenoscope elevator region with magnifying glasses has been proposed to identify damage.[33] Additionally, over the past 2 years, studies have used borescope inspection of endoscope working channels to identify internal damage within these endoscope channels. These studies have been conducted at ambulatory surgery centers[34,35] and academic tertiary care institutions.[36,37] Initial studies performed at an ambulatory surgery center reported widespread channel damage and debris within endoscope working channels,[34,35] with a cumulative increase in the amount of adherent debris over a 7-month observation period.[35] These concerning findings necessitated sending the majority of endoscopes at the facility for repairs.[34,35] Subsequent studies from tertiary academic centers were more reassuring, reporting predominantly mild expected "wear and tear" damage within the majority of endoscopes in use.[36,37] Damage rating scales have been proposed in these studies and one of these rating systems[36] has been successfully used in subsequent studies to evaluate the impact of endoscope working channel damage on endoscope reprocessing and residue after reprocessing.[25,36,38]

Overall, these studies have highlighted the issue of endoscope working channel damage. Although mild wear and tear working channel damage is unlikely to affect the adequacy of reprocessing, more severe damage may well do so. The extent to which accumulated endoscope working channel damage renders an endoscope "unusable" requires further study; however, a threshold of working channel damage above which an endoscope becomes high risk for infection transmission may be identified and characterized. Current consensus and practice for endoscope maintenance is for adherence to manufacturer-recommended endoscope maintenance protocols, with periodic replacement of elements of the endoscopes that are exposed to increased mechanical stress or use. Some investigators have proposed the inclusion of routine borescope examination of endoscope channels as a part of standard reprocessing. However, the validity of this approach requires further study.

NOVEL ALGORITHMS FOR REPROCESSING ENDOSCOPES
Double Reprocessing

Double reprocessing has primarily been studied in duodenoscopes and linear echoendoscopes, because these endoscopes with an elevator mechanism carry the highest risk for transmission of infection.[11] In a study published in 2017, we demonstrated a beneficial role of 2 full cycles of duodenoscope reprocessing in reducing bioburden.[11] Compared with duodenoscopes that had only undergone 1 cycle of reprocessing, duodenoscopes subjected to 2 cycles of all elements of reprocessing including precleaning, manual cleaning and HLD exhibited a significant decrease in postreprocessing elevator channel bioburden as measured by ATP bioluminescence.[11]

However, a prospective randomized study performed in a nonoutbreak setting using bacterial culture-based assessments, found no significant difference between single and double HLD with regard to the proportion of duodenoscopes that were culture positive for 10 or more colony-forming units (CFU) (2.3% vs 4.1%) or greater than 0 CFU (16.1% vs 16.0%) growth of any aerobic bacteria.[39] Notably, duodenoscopes in the double HLD limb of the study underwent only a single round of manual cleaning.

A subsequent prospective randomized study of duodenoscopes and linear echoendoscopes also demonstrated no benefit of dual cycles of endoscope reprocessing.[40] This prospective randomized study included 4 centers and evaluated 5850 surveillance culture specimens obtained during 2925 encounters from 45 duodenoscopes and linear echoendoscopes in clinical use. The study found that double HLD of duodenoscopes and linear echoendoscopes did not decrease culture positivity rates compared with single HLD in any of the 4 facilities.[40] Among the 224 encounters with positive growth, 140 microbes (62.5%) originated from samples collected from the elevator mechanism, 73 (32.6%) originated from samples collected from the channel, and 11 (4.9%) originated from both samples.[40] High concern organisms were only detected in 8 specimens (0.1%). There was no statistically significant difference between single and double HLD ($P>.05$ for all comparisons).[40] However, this study was underpowered to detect differences in the impact of single versus double HLD on culture rates for high concern pathogens, and the culture methods used may have been insensitive. Again, only the HLD step was repeated in this study, and not the precleaning and manual cleaning steps.

Finally, a further study evaluated culture positivity rates after 2 full cycles of manual cleaning and HLD.[41] This study found that modification in the precleaning fluid and use of an FDA-recommended cleaning brush was associated with a decrease in culture positivity rates from 9.4% (0.8% rate of known pathogens) in 627 cultures to 4.8% (0.2% rate of known pathogens) in 420 cultures.[41] A primary conclusion of this study was that double HLD resulted in a low rate of positive cultures for known pathogens and for organisms of low pathogenic potential, but did not eliminate these positive cultures.[41] This conclusion is reasonable and would be supported by many.

Variability in the definition of double HLD—with some studies defining double HLD as repetition of all steps in cleaning (including precleaning and manual cleaning)[11,40] and others defining double HLD as repetition of only HLD/AER cycles after a single cycle of precleaning and manual cleaning,[39] enhances challenges associated with comparison of these approaches, as does institutional variability in baseline culture positivity rates. It is also worth noting that, in the culture and quarantine approach discussed elsewhere in this article, positive cultures are typically managed by 1 or more repeat cycles of manual cleaning and HLD, usually with limination of the previously cultured bacteria.[42] This process is arguably analogous to double HLD.

Nevertheless, despite the mixed data in nonoutbreak settings, a survey study evaluating practice patterns for duodenoscope reprocessing found that double HLD was the most common enhanced reprocessing technique used by responding institutions (63.1% of centers).[43] This finding is not surprising, because this approach offers the advantages of ease and convenience and does not require hiring of additional personnel, the establishment of additional institutional infrastructure, or the purchase of additional duodenoscopes. Moreover, it is easily combined with additional enhanced reprocessing techniques, such as a shift to liquid chemical sterilization.

Culture and Quarantine

Culture and quarantine/hold protocols have been shown to be useful in the setting of recent outbreaks of infection related to duodenoscopes.[7,8] Investigations at some centers where outbreaks occurred revealed that the centers were largely following established duodenoscope reprocessing guidelines for HLD.[28,32] Indeed, at one of the centers with a reported outbreak, 3% of duodenoscope cultures continued to be positive despite careful cleaning and HLD of duodenoscopes.[32] In these high-risk scenarios, endoscope culture and hold protocols are valuable in detecting persistent contamination of duodenoscopes and in removal from use of duodenoscopes with persistent culture positivity.[8] Persistent culture positivity may be related to undiagnosed internal damage to the duodenoscopes.[42]

The culture and quarantine approach is a stringent protocol in which all duodenoscopes are cultured after each reprocessing cycle and held in "quarantine" until they are confirmed to be culture negative.[44] If cultures return positive, the duodenoscope undergoes repeat reprocessing and is then recultured. Once culture negativity is established, a further cycle of reprocessing is undertaken before the duodenoscope is released for patient use. This approach is thorough and may potentially prevent transmission of infection related to duodenoscopes, if cultures are assumed to be accurate and reliable. However, the approach may be less practical at institutions with a high procedural volume and a limited number of duodenoscopes, because a given duodenoscope may be out of use for up to 3 days while culture results are awaited. Implementing such a strategy successfully requires investment in equipment, staffing, and infrastructure. A substantial (approximately 3-fold) increase in the number of duodenoscopes in circulation would be necessary for implementation of this protocol at an institution, together with an expansion of endoscope storage capacity. Additional staff numbers and training will be necessary for carrying out duodenal sampling for cultures and the additional cycle of reprocessing. Finally, an institutional microbiology infrastructure will need to be established for performing duodenoscope cultures. In an outbreak setting, a culture and hold strategy is essential. However, in nonoutbreak settings some investigators have proposed limiting costs by culturing only a rotating proportion of duodenoscopes after use, ensuring that all duodenoscopes get cultured over a preset period of time.[45,46]

Endoscope Sterilization

The inherent composition and design of endoscopes prevents them from being autoclaving for sterilization. Alternative lower temperature sterilization processes have been proposed and used for endoscope sterilization, including ethylene oxide (EtO) gas sterilization, hydrogen peroxide gas sterilization, per-acetic acid sterilization, and low temperature steam and formaldehyde sterilization.

Interest was generated in the use of EtO as a modality for duodenoscope sterilization after an initial report of termination of an outbreak of multidrug-resistant organisms (MDRO) after change in institutional reprocessing practice from HLD to sterilization with EtO.[28] When EtO sterilization is undertaken, this usually occurs at offsite facilities. Initial steps in the process, therefore, include transport to the sterilization facility and then back to the hospital for use, in addition to the time necessary for duodenoscope sterilization. This process results in the unavailability of the endoscope for 2 to 3 days and thus the need for approximately 2- to 3-fold more duodenoscopes in circulation at the facility. Furthermore, EtO sterilization tends to cause more damage to endoscopes,[47] and is thought to decrease the lifespan of endoscopes relative to standard endoscope reprocessing, which may require more frequent duodenoscope replacement. These factors result in not insubstantial costs, and it has been estimated that a shift to EtO would increase the cost of each endoscopic retrograde cholangiopancreatography by $1043.[48] Finally, concerns exist over its potential carcinogenicity and other occupational hazards.[49] These many issues have led to limited institutional adoption of EtO sterilization, with a survey study indicating adoption by just 12% of responding institutions.[43] Moreover, there is lack of clear evidence indicating superiority of EtO sterilization over standard reprocessing in nonoutbreak settings. A prospective randomized study comparing single HLD, double HLD, and HLD followed by EtO in a nonoutbreak setting, found no difference between these approaches with regards to the proportion of duodenoscopes that were culture positive with 10 or more CFU (2.3% vs 4.1% vs 4.2%) or more than 0 CFU (16.1% vs 16% vs 22.5%) growth of aerobic bacteria.[39] Additionally, a recent publication from a center with a previously described outbreak demonstrated a 1.2% positive culture rate for carbapenem-resistant *Enterobacteriaceae* from duodenoscopes even after EtO sterilization.[47]

In a recent study, EtO sterilization was undertaken in a targeted manner. To identify specific procedures after which EtO sterilization should occur, patients were administered preprocedure risk stratification questionnaires, asked to undergo CRE polymerase chain reaction screening for MDRO presences from a rectal swab, and procedures were evaluated for the presence of purulent cholangitis or infected pancreatic fluid collections.[50] Based on these criteria, 2 endoscopes per week underwent EtO sterilization on a rotating basis. Although larger patient sample sizes and multi-institutional studies would be informative, this initial study of targeted EtO sterilization after duodenoscope use in the highest risk patients was notable for elimination of endoscope-associated MDRO transmission at the institution in which the study was conducted.[50]

Owing to concerns and technical limitations, as well as limited data supporting its efficacy, EtO sterilization is not practical at many ambulatory centers and academic institutions that perform high-volume endoscopy in the setting of relative resource restriction resulting in a limited number inventory of endoscopes/duodenoscopes. EtO sterilization has anecdotally been effective in terminating outbreaks at centers where it has been used,[28,30] and will therefore likely continue to be used in outbreak settings or at institutions with a high prevalence of MDRO. However, screening of individuals for MDRO colonization/infection before endoscopic retrograde cholangiopancreatography and targeted sterilization of endoscopes after use in these patients with MDROs might be a reasonable potential approach for minimizing infection transmission.

Liquid chemical sterilization

Although EtO-based sterilization is most common, other sterilization approaches are in practice as well. For example, an automated approach for using per-acetic acid to achieve chemical sterilization was first introduced in 1988 and has been used for some medical, dental and surgical instruments within the United States.[51,52] Some chemical agents and solutions are cleared for use in HLD and may be used for liquid chemical sterilization by extending the duration of exposure based on simulated use testing with spores.[53] This liquid chemical sterilization approach has associated limitations of lower penetration capability and nonlinear bactericidal kinetics, but the FDA has offered this approach as an option for enhanced duodenoscope reprocessing.[53] Two AERs have been cleared as liquid chemical sterilant processing systems, both of which are manufactured by the STERIS Corporation (Mentor, OH).[53] These AER systems expose the device surfaces and lumens to a liquid chemical sterilant and then rinse the duodenoscope with extensively treated or filtered water.[53] A recent duodenoscope reprocessing survey indicated that 34.5% of responding institutions have adopted this approach.[43]

ENDOSCOPE DRYING

Drying is increasingly recognized as an important element of endoscope reprocessing, because residual fluid within endoscope working channels after reprocessing may promote the growth of pathogens.[54,55] Drying of endoscope working channels has traditionally been a manually performed process, one that is subject to human lapses. Current multisociety reprocessing guidelines recommend endoscope drying with administration of forced filtered air; however, there are no specific recommendations regarding the duration of air drying or the modality by which it is administered.[4]

Data regarding the necessity of, and optimal modalities for, the drying of flexible endoscopes after reprocessing are limited, and recommendations from different sources are variable and sometimes conflicting. For example, alcohol flushes before and after drying are recommended by some for their antimicrobial activity[56] and to promote drying.[4,57,58] In contrast, the British Society of Gastroenterology recommends against alcohol flushes owing to concerns that the fixative properties of alcohol may, over time, promote pathogen retention and accumulation within endoscopes.[59,60] Similarly, although the Association of perioperative Registered Nurses emphasizes the importance of uniformly following and enforcing practices that ensure thorough drying of endoscopes after each reprocessing cycle to prevent transmission of infection,[61] other groups and societies such as the British Society of Gastroenterology and the Steering Group for Flexible Endoscope Cleaning and Disinfection have suggested that drying may not be as important if an endoscope is used within 3 to 4 hours of HLD.[60,62] Gastroenterology societies that have commented on this issue, uniformly support the importance of thorough drying if longer term storage of endoscopes is planned.[5,60–62]

Perhaps as a consequence of these conflicting recommendations, endoscope reprocessing, drying, and storage practices are highly variable among institutions and inadequate approaches may result in retained fluid, bioburden, and biofilm formation. In a recent duodenoscope reprocessing survey, only 47.8% of the 249 responding centers reported using the AER air purge cycle, or any postprocessing drying practice such as administration of manual forced air to the working channel.[43]

In a recent study of drying and storage practices at 3 hospitals, visual examinations and tests to detect fluid and microbial contamination within endoscope working channels were conducted on patient-ready endoscopes.[63] Importantly, residual fluid was detected in the working channels of 49% of these endoscopes, all of which had been stored for at least 24 hours and were deemed ready for patient use.[63] In addition to, or perhaps as a consequence of, residual fluid detected within endoscope working channels, residual bioburden was detected by ATP testing in 22% of these endoscopes.[63] Endoscope culture protocols were also used in this study and the presence of residual bioburden significantly correlated with retained moisture. Microbial growth was detected in 71% of endoscopes.[63] These findings make a compelling argument that insufficient drying contributes to retained fluid and microbial contamination within endoscope working channels.

Our group recently performed a systematic study comparing manual and automated drying. This study revealed that automated drying is significantly more effective than manual drying in eliminating fluid from endoscope working channels.[38] Automated administration of filtered air at controlled pressure through all internal endoscope channels using a device (DriScope Aid) resulted in significantly fewer fluid droplets compared with manual drying.[38] Additionally, lower levels of retained bioburden were present after automated drying, as evidenced by lower working channel ATP bioluminescence values 48 hours after drying.[38] Notably, there was virtually no retained fluid evident within endoscope working channels after automated drying for 10 minutes.[38] These findings support recommendations for automation of as many reprocessing steps as possible, and confirm that automated drying may decrease the risk of transmission of infection related to endoscopy.

ENDOSCOPE STORAGE

Fluid within endoscope working channels diminishes over time when endoscopes are hung vertically in air circulation or drying cabinets.[64,65] Consistent with this practice, a recent endoscope drying study demonstrated fewer working channel fluid droplets at sequential time points in the 72 hours after manual drying.[38] Endoscope working channels had significantly lower ATP bioluminescence values after 48 and 72 hours of endoscope hang time after automated drying, in comparison with manual drying.[38] Elevated ATP bioluminescence values may reflect bacterial proliferation in residual moisture that remains within endoscope working channels after manual drying. Furthermore, after automated drying, there was no significant difference in working channel fluid droplets between endoscopes that were stored vertically and those that were stored horizontally, coiled in compact transport bins, suggesting that storage modality may be less important if endoscopes are thoroughly dried before storage.

Gastroenterology society guidelines recommend the use of endoscopes within 5 to 7 days of reprocessing.[4] Endoscopes should be stored in a ventilated, dust-free cabinet. Limited data support the safety of using endoscopes within 21 days after reprocessing if they are appropriately stored.[65] The potential safety of 21-day endoscope storage is based on a prospective observational study in a tertiary care center that evaluated a limited number of duodenoscopes, colonoscopes, and gastroscopes by culturing endoscopes at 0, 7, 12, and 14 days after reprocessing. Although there were 33 positive cultures of the 96 cultures obtained (29.2% overall contamination rate), 29 of the 33 bacterial cultured were typical skin or environmental contaminants and were determined to be clinically insignificant.[65] Four potential pathogens were cultured (Candida, Enterococcus, Streptococcus, and Aureobasidium) and all reportedly grew at low concentrations.[65] However, the optimal and acceptable intervals between reprocessing and use remain uncertain and in need of further study. The acceptable storage interval for gastrointestinal endoscopes before use has a substantial impact on endoscopy unit workflow and productivity.

The identification of optimal endoscope storage conditions has been the topic of several studies, the most recent of which assessed the efficacy of an automated drying and storage cabinet compared with a standard storage cabinet in achieving endoscope dryness after reprocessing and in decreasing the risk of microbial growth.[55] The automated cabinet was found to be advantageous for rapid drying of endoscope surfaces and in reducing the risk of microbial growth after reprocessing.[55] In this study, drying times of bronchoscopes, colonoscopes, and duodenoscopes were measured using each cabinet. With use of the automated drying and storage cabinet, internal endoscope channels were dry at 1 hour and external surfaces after 3 hours of storage. By comparison, for endoscopes that were stored in the standard storage cabinet, residual internal fluid was detected within endoscope working channels after 24 hours of storage.[55] Similar to, and as an extension of, the advantages of automated drying of endoscope working channels, automated drying within endoscope storage cabinets seems to be advantages in creating an inner working channel environment devoid of the fluid residue sanctuary for microbes.

SUMMARY

In this era of enhanced scrutiny after outbreaks of duodenoscope-transmitted infection with MDRO, it has become increasingly clear that institutions must optimize their endoscope reprocessing programs. There is increasing recognition that standard endoscope reprocessing practices may not represent the ideal approach for preventing transmission of infection related to endoscopy. In this article, we have discussed multiple approaches to enhance and optimize reprocessing, drying, and storage of standard duodenoscopes. The optimal enhanced duodenoscope reprocessing modality remains to be determined and is an area in need of further research. In the absence of definitive data, and while anticipating the eventual availability of additional data and guidelines, each institution must decide which approach(es) to surveillance and enhanced duodenoscope reprocessing are most appropriate locally, based on the procedure volume, the background MDRO infection rates at the institution and on institutional budgetary constraints. Acknowledging the challenges and limitations in effectively reprocessing duodenoscopes, the FDA in August 2019 issued a safety communiqué recommending transitioning to either single use disposable duodenoscopes, or to duodenoscopes with innovative designs that allow more effective reprocessing, such as duodenoscopes with detachable disposable endcaps or entirely disposable distal tips, which include the elevator.[18]

DISCLOSURE

None of the authors have any conflicts of interest pertaining to the study to disclose.

REFERENCES

1. Spaulding EH. Chemical disinfection of medical and surgical materials. In: Block SS, editor. Disinfection S, and Preservation. Lawrence (CA): Lea and Febiger; 1968. p. 517.

2. Committee AQAIE, Petersen BT, Chennat J, et al. Multisociety guideline on reprocessing flexible gastrointestinal endoscopes: 2011. Gastrointest Endosc 2011;73:1075–84.

3. Rutala WA, Kanamori H, Sickbert-Bennett EE, et al. What's new in reprocessing endoscopes: are we going to ensure "the needs of the patient come first" by shifting from disinfection to sterilization? Am J Infect Control 2019;47S:A62–6.

4. Reprocessing Guideline Task Force, Petersen BT, Cohen J, et al. Multisociety guideline on reprocessing flexible GI endoscopes: 2016 update. Gastrointest Endosc 2017;85:282–294 e1.

5. Committee AT, Komanduri S, Abu Dayyeh BK, et al. Technologies for monitoring the quality of endoscope reprocessing. Gastrointest Endosc 2014;80:369–73.

6. Cori L, Ofstead MMRQ, Eiland JE, et al. CRCST. A glimpse at the true cost of reprocessing endoscopes. 2016. Available at: www.iahcsmm.org. Accessed March 21, 2020.

7. Chiu KW, Fong TV, Wu KL, et al. Surveillance culture of endoscope to monitor the quality of high-level disinfection of gastrointestinal reprocessing. Hepatogastroenterology 2010;57:531–4.

8. Higa JT, Choe J, Tombs D, et al. Optimizing duodenoscope reprocessing: rigorous assessment of a culture and quarantine protocol. Gastrointest Endosc 2018;88:223–9.

9. Lu LS, Wu KL, Chiu YC, et al. Swab culture monitoring of automated endoscope reprocessors after high-level disinfection. World J Gastroenterol 2012;18:1660–3.

10. Hansen D, Benner D, Hilgenhoner M, et al. ATP measurement as method to monitor the quality of reprocessing flexible endoscopes. Ger Med Sci 2004;2: Doc04.

11. Sethi S, Huang RJ, Barakat MT, et al. Adenosine triphosphate bioluminescence for bacteriologic surveillance and reprocessing strategies for minimizing risk of infection transmission by duodenoscopes. Gastrointest Endosc 2017;85: 1180–1187 e1.

12. Bommarito M, Stahl J, Morse D, et al. Monitoring the efficacy of the cleaning and disinfection process for flexible endoscopes by quantification of multiple biological markers. Antimicrob Resist Infect Control 2015;4:P56.

13. Parohl N, Stiefenhofer D, Heiligtag S, et al. Monitoring of endoscope reprocessing with an adenosine triphosphate (ATP) bioluminescence method. GMS Hyg Infect Control 2017;12:Doc04.

14. Visrodia K, Hanada Y, Pennington KM, et al. Duodenoscope reprocessing surveillance with adenosine triphosphate testing and terminal cultures: a clinical pilot study. Gastrointest Endosc 2017;86:180–6.

15. Quan E, Mahmood R, Naik A, et al. Use of adenosine triphosphate to audit reprocessing of flexible endoscopes with an elevator mechanism. Am J Infect Control 2018;46:1272–7.

16. Alfa MJ, Fatima I, Olson N. The adenosine triphosphate test is a rapid and reliable audit tool to assess manual cleaning adequacy of flexible endoscope channels. Am J Infect Control 2013;41:249–53.

17. Turner DE, Daugherity EK, Altier C, et al. Efficacy and limitations of an ATP-based monitoring system. J Am Assoc Lab Anim Sci 2010;49:190–5.

18. Administration TUSFaD. The FDA is recommending transition to duodenoscopes with innovative designs to enhance safety. Safety Communication; 2019. Available at: https://www.fda.gov/medical-devices/safety-communications/fda-recommending-transition-duodenoscopes-innovative-designs-enhance-safety-fda-safety-communication. Accessed April 25, 2020.

19. Alfa MJ, Olson N, Degagne P, et al. Development and validation of rapid use scope test strips to determine the efficacy of manual cleaning for flexible endoscope channels. Am J Infect Control 2012;40:860–5.

20. Beilenhoff U, Neumann CS, Biering H, et al. ESGE/ESGENA guideline for process validation and routine testing for reprocessing endoscopes in washer-disinfectors, according to the European Standard prEN ISO 15883 parts 1, 4 and 5. Endoscopy 2007;39:85–94.

21. Beilenhoff U, Neumann CS, Rey JF, et al. ESGE-ESGENA guideline for quality assurance in reprocessing: microbiological surveillance testing in endoscopy. Endoscopy 2007;39:175–81.

22. Collaboration DoHaHS. Duodenoscope Surveillance Sampling & Culturing. 2018:1-58. Available at: https://www.fda.gov/media/111081/download. Accessed April 25, 2020.

23. Ofstead CL, Wetzler HP, Snyder AK, et al. Endoscope reprocessing methods: a prospective study on the impact of human factors and automation. Gastroenterol Nurs 2010;33:304–11.

24. Rutala WA, Weber DJ. Healthcare Infection Control Practices Advisory Committee. Guidelines for disinfection and sterilization in healthcare facilities. Available at: https://www.cdc.gov/infectioncontrol/pdf/guidelines/disinfection-guidelines 2008. Accessed March 21, 2020.

25. Barakat MT, Huang RJ, Banerjee S. Simethicone is retained in endoscopes despite reprocessing: impact of its use on working channel fluid retention and adenosine triphosphate bioluminescence values (with video). Gastrointest Endosc 2019;89:115–23.

26. Ofstead CL, Wetzler HP, Johnson EA, et al. Simethicone residue remains inside gastrointestinal endoscopes despite reprocessing. Am J Infect Control 2016; 44:1237–40.

27. van Stiphout SH, Laros IF, van Wezel RA, et al. Crystallization in the waterjet channel in colonoscopes due to simethicone. Endoscopy 2016;48:E394–5.

28. Epstein L, Hunter JC, Arwady MA, et al. New Delhi metallo-beta-lactamase-producing carbapenem-resistant Escherichia coli associated with exposure to duodenoscopes. JAMA 2014;312:1447–55.

29. Kola A, Piening B, Pape UF, et al. An outbreak of carbapenem-resistant OXA-48 - producing Klebsiella pneumonia associated to duodenoscopy. Antimicrob Resist Infect Control 2015;4:8.

30. Smith ZL, Oh YS, Saeian K, et al. Transmission of carbapenem-resistant Enterobacteriaceae during ERCP: time to revisit the current reprocessing guidelines. Gastrointest Endosc 2015;81:1041–5.

31. Verfaillie CJ, Bruno MJ, Voor in 't Holt AF, et al. Withdrawal of a novel-design duodenoscope ends outbreak of a VIM-2-producing Pseudomonas aeruginosa. Endoscopy 2015;47:493–502.

32. Wendorf KA, Kay M, Baliga C, et al. Endoscopic retrograde cholangiopancreatography-associated AmpC Escherichia coli outbreak. Infect Control Hosp Epidemiol 2015;36:634–42.

33. Beilenhoff U, Biering H, Blum R, et al. Reprocessing of flexible endoscopes and endoscopic accessories used in gastrointestinal endoscopy: Position Statement of the European Society of Gastrointestinal Endoscopy (ESGE) and European Society of Gastroenterology Nurses and Associates (ESGENA) - Update 2018. Endoscopy 2018;50:1205–34.

34. Ofstead CL, Wetzler HP, Eiland JE, et al. Assessing residual contamination and damage inside flexible endoscopes over time. Am J Infect Control 2016;44: 1675–7.

35. Ofstead CL, Wetzler HP, Heymann OL, et al. Longitudinal assessment of reprocessing effectiveness for colonoscopes and gastroscopes: results of visual

inspections, biochemical markers, and microbial cultures. Am J Infect Control 2017;45:e26–33.

36. Barakat MT, Girotra M, Huang RJ, et al. Scoping the scope: endoscopic evaluation of endoscope working channels with a new high-resolution inspection endoscope (with video). Gastrointest Endosc 2018;88:601–611 e1.

37. Thaker AM, Kim S, Sedarat A, et al. Inspection of endoscope instrument channels after reprocessing using a prototype borescope. Gastrointest Endosc 2018;88: 612–9.

38. Barakat MT, Huang RJ, Banerjee S. Comparison of automated and manual drying in the elimination of residual endoscope working channel fluid after reprocessing (with video). Gastrointest Endosc 2019;89:124–132 e2.

39. Snyder GM, Wright SB, Smithey A, et al. Randomized Comparison of 3 High-Level Disinfection and Sterilization Procedures for Duodenoscopes. Gastroenterology 2017;153:1018–25.

40. Bartles RL, Leggett JE, Hove S, et al. A randomized trial of single versus double high-level disinfection of duodenoscopes and linear echoendoscopes using standard automated reprocessing. Gastrointest Endosc 2018;88: 306–313 e2.

41. Rex DK, Sieber M, Lehman GA, et al. A double-reprocessing high-level disinfection protocol does not eliminate positive cultures from the elevators of duodenoscopes. Endoscopy 2018;50:588–96.

42. Mark JA, Underberg K, Kramer RE. Results of duodenoscope culture and quarantine after manufacturer-recommended cleaning process. Gastrointest Endosc 2020;91(6):1328–33.

43. Thaker AM, Muthusamy VR, Sedarat A, et al. Duodenoscope reprocessing practice patterns in U.S. endoscopy centers: a survey study. Gastrointest Endosc 2018;88:316–322 e2.

44. Ross AS, Baliga C, Verma P, et al. A quarantine process for the resolution of duodenoscope-associated transmission of multidrug-resistant Escherichia coli. Gastrointest Endosc 2015;82:477–83.

45. Beilenhoff U, Biering H, Blum R, et al. Prevention of multidrug-resistant infections from contaminated duodenoscopes: Position Statement of the European Society of Gastrointestinal Endoscopy (ESGE) and European Society of Gastroenterology Nurses and Associates (ESGENA). Endoscopy 2017;49:1098–106.

46. Rutala WA, Weber DJ. ERCP scopes: what can we do to prevent infections? Infect Control Hosp Epidemiol 2015;36:643–8.

47. Naryzhny I, Silas D, Chi K. Impact of ethylene oxide gas sterilization of duodenoscopes after a carbapenem-resistant Enterobacteriaceae outbreak. Gastrointest Endosc 2016;84:259–62.

48. Almario CV, May FP, Shaheen NJ, et al. Cost utility of competing strategies to prevent endoscopic transmission of carbapenem-resistant enterobacteriaceae. Am J Gastroenterol 2015;110:1666–74.

49. IARC eCAaROARoHCFeL, France; 2012. Available at: https://monographs.iarc.fr/wp-content/uploads/2018/06/mono100F-28.pdf. Accessed April 25, 2020.

50. Smith ZL, Dua A, Saeian K, et al. A novel protocol obviates endoscope sampling for carbapenem-resistant enterobacteriaceae: experience of a center with a prior outbreak. Dig Dis Sci 2017;62:3100–9.

51. Chenjiao W, Hongyan Z, Qing G, et al. In-use evaluation of peracetic acid for high-level disinfection of endoscopes. Gastroenterol Nurs 2016;39: 116–20.

52. Cheung RJ, Ortiz D, DiMarino AJ Jr. GI endoscopic reprocessing practices in the United States. Gastrointest Endosc 1999;50:362–8.

53. Administration UFaD. Reducing the Risk of Infection from Reprocessed Duodenoscopes. November 6-7, 2019 meeting of the General Hospital and Personal Use Devices Panel of the Medical Devices Advisory Committee 2019.

54. Alfa MJ, Sitter DL. In-hospital evaluation of contamination of duodenoscopes: a quantitative assessment of the effect of drying. J Hosp Infect 1991;19: 89–98.

55. Perumpail RB, Marya NB, McGinty BL, et al. Endoscope reprocessing: comparison of drying effectiveness and microbial levels with an automated drying and storage cabinet with forced filtered air and a standard storage cabinet. Am J Infect Control 2019;47(9):1083–9.

56. McDonnell G, Russell AD. Antiseptics and disinfectants: activity, action, and resistance. Clin Microbiol Rev 1999;12:147–79.

57. Nelson DB, Muscarella LF. Current issues in endoscope reprocessing and infection control during gastrointestinal endoscopy. World J Gastroenterol 2006;12: 3953–64.

58. Asge Standards Of Practice C, Banerjee S, Shen B, et al. Infection control during GI endoscopy. Gastrointest Endosc 2008;67:781–90.

59. Beilenhoff U, Neumann CS, Rey JF, et al. ESGE-ESGENA Guideline: cleaning and disinfection in gastrointestinal endoscopy. Endoscopy 2008;40:939–57.

60. Gastroenterology BSo. British Society of Gastroenterology Guidelines for decontamination of equipment for gastrointestinal endoscopy. Available at: http://www.bsg.org.uk/images/stories/docs/clinical/guidelines/endoscopy/decontamination_2014_v2.pdf 2014. Accessed March 21, 2020.

61. AORN. Guideline at a glance: processing flexible endoscopes. AORN J 2016; 104:610–5.

62. (SFERD). Steering Group for Flexible Endoscope Cleaning and Disinfection. Professional Standard Handbook. Flexible Endoscope Cleaning and Disinfection. Available at: http://wfhss.com/wp-content/uploads/SFERD-Professional-Standard-Handbook-3-1-UK-definitief.pdf 2014. Accessed March 21, 2020.

63. Ofstead CL, Heymann OL, Quick MR, et al. Residual moisture and waterborne pathogens inside flexible endoscopes: evidence from a multisite study of endoscope drying effectiveness. Am J Infect Control 2018;46:689–96.

64. Pineau L, Villard E, Duc DL, et al. Endoscope drying/storage cabinet: interest and efficacy. J Hosp Infect 2008;68:59–65.

65. Brock AS, Steed LL, Freeman J, et al. Endoscope storage time: assessment of microbial colonization up to 21 days after reprocessing. Gastrointest Endosc 2015;81:1150–4.

Quality Systems Approach for Endoscope Reprocessing
You Don't Know What You Don't Know!

Michelle J. Alfa, PhD, FCCM

KEYWORDS

- Cleaning monitoring • Wet storage • Humidicator test • Rapid cleaning tests
- Human factors • Duodenoscopes • Borescopes

KEY POINTS

- Currently, there is little monitoring of the various stages in endoscope reprocessing, so most endoscopy clinics do not know if they have problems.
- Monitoring of manual cleaning efficacy is crucial to ensure ongoing compliance of reprocessing personnel.
- Monitoring of moisture in endoscope channels in storage is crucial to ensure dry storage, thereby preventing microbial replication that could lead to biofilm or buildup biofilm formation.
- Monitoring for microbial contamination in patient-ready endoscopes requires culture and cannot be achieved using rapid adenosine triphosphate tests.
- Implementation of a quality management system specific for endoscope reprocessing is crucial and needs to include monitoring and documentation of ongoing compliance.

INTRODUCTION

The infection outbreaks attributable to contaminated endoscopes have been reviewed in prior articles. These outbreaks involved many types of endoscopes (eg, bronchoscopes, cystoscopes, duodenoscopes, gastroscopes, and colonoscopes) and often were identified because they involved transmission of multidrug-resistant organisms. In addition, the postmarket clinical study initiated by the US Food and Drug Administration (FDA) in 2015[1] required the 3 main duodenoscope manufacturers (ie, Olympus, Pentax, and Fujinon) to undertake culture monitoring post–high-level disinfection (HLD) to better understand the existing contamination rates in clinically used duodenoscopes. The 2019 interim FDA statement[2] reported that 5.4% of fully reprocessed duodenoscopes were contaminated with high-concern organisms and that an additional 3.6% were contaminated with low to moderate organisms. The FDA interim report[2] on this most recent data indicated that they expected contamination rates

Department of Medical Microbiology, University of Manitoba, Winnipeg, Manitoba, Canada
E-mail address: michellealfa001@gmail.com

Gastrointest Endoscopy Clin N Am 30 (2020) 693–709
https://doi.org/10.1016/j.giec.2020.06.005
1052-5157/20/© 2020 Elsevier Inc. All rights reserved.

to be less than 1% and the level of contamination detected in duodenoscopes "… shows that improvements are necessary…". They mention the need to improve cleaning and to explore whether meticulous cleaning combined with sterilization might offer a more effective option. In the most recent August 29, 2019, FDA safety communication,[3] the recommendations include a transition away from fixed endcap duodenoscopes to those that have disposable or removable endcaps or other new design features that eliminate or facilitate reprocessing. They also recommended that endoscopy sites institute quality assurance programs that utilize sample and culture of duodenoscopes and other monitoring methods. Without monitoring of the critical stages in reprocessing (manual cleaning stage, dry storage, viable organisms post-HLD, and so forth), endoscopy clinics cannot truly identify what needs to change and then document monitoring data to confirm the impact of any changes implemented.

> In terms of reprocessing of flexible endoscopes - endoscopy clinics cannot keep doing the same things and expect a different outcome. The key question is, "What needs to change?" It is difficult to identify effective changes in endoscope reprocessing because currently there is no monitoring being performed!

MONITORING CRITICAL STAGES IN ENDOSCOPE REPROCESSING

For reprocessing of surgical devices, there is extensive monitoring outlined in reprocessing guidelines that includes weekly (preferably daily) monitoring of the cleaning efficacy of the washer-disinfector and the use of biological and chemical indicators for the steam sterilized packages as well as review and sign-off on printouts to monitor and confirm the adequacy of each steam sterilizer cycle.[4,5] There are similar requirements for low-temperature sterilization processes. The recent review by Alfa and Singh[6] summarized endoscope reprocessing guidelines and indicated that the monitoring for endoscope reprocessing was highly variable between countries (**Table 1**).[7–17] This summary of guideline requirements identifies some of the disconnects in endoscope reprocessing, such as the lack of recommendations regarding the following:

- The impact of simethicone, tissue glue, dyes, and so forth used during clinical endoscopic procedures on the efficacy of endoscope channel cleaning
- The efficacy of manual cleaning of endoscope channels prior to HLD
- The extent of channel drying needed to ensure moisture is not present during storage.
- The use of culture to evaluate microbial contamination in channels of patient-ready endoscopes

Because monitoring of many of the critical issues in endoscopy reprocessing is not required by North American reprocessing guidelines[9–12] nor is it required of manufacturers validation of cleaning instructions,[18,19] it means that endoscopy clinics in North America (large and small) do not perform much monitoring and as such they do not know how well or how poorly they are doing with respect to many of these disconnect issues (ie, "you don't know what you don't know").

MONITORING MANUAL CLEANING EFFICACY

The bedside clean after a patient procedure is important to ensure that gross debris is immediately flushed from the endoscope channels. This reduces the risk that patient-derived residuals dry in the channels or on the exterior of the endoscope during transit

Table 1
Current endoscope reprocessing recommendations from guidelines

Guideline[a]	Simethicone, Dye, or Glue Used for Patient Procedure	Transit Time from Patient Procedure to Start of Reprocessing	Manual or Automated Endoscope Reprocessor Cleaning and Rinsing	Monitoring of Manual Cleaning	High-Level Disinfection[d] or Sterilization	MEC Testing	Alcohol Flush and Dry	Storage	Monitoring of Residual Moisture	Culture of Endoscopes and Automated Endoscope Reprocessor
Canada[b]										
PIDAC, 2016[7]	N/A	Yes	Manual ± AER[c]	Yes	Either, GI scopes HLD	Yes	Yes	Regular cabinet	No	Outbreak only
Health Canada, 2010[8]	N/A		Manual or AER[c]	Yes	Either, GI scopes HLD	Yes	Yes	Regular or channel-purge cabinet	No	No
USA										
SGNA, 2015[9]	N/A		Manual ± AER[c]	N/A	Either, GI scopes HLD	Yes	Yes[e]	Regular cabinet	No	No
ANSI/AAMI ST91:2015[10]	N/A		Manual + AER[c]	Yes	Either, GI scopes HLD	Yes	Yes[e]	Regular cabinet or channel-purge cabinet	No	No
Multisociety; Petersen, 2017[11]	N/A		Manual + AER[c]	N/A	Either, GI scopes HLD	N/A	Yes	Regular cabinet	No	No
ASGE; Calderwood, 2018[12]	N/A		Manual	N/A	Either, GI scopes HLD	YES	Yes	Regular cabinet	No	No

(continued on next page)

Table 1
(continued)

Guideline[a]	Simethicone, Dye, or Glue Used for Patient Procedure	Transit Time from Patient Procedure to Start of Reprocessing	Manual or Automated Endoscope Reprocessor Cleaning and Rinsing	Monitoring of Manual Cleaning	High-Level Disinfection[d] or Sterilization	MEC Testing	Alcohol Flush and Dry	Storage	Monitoring of Residual Moisture	Culture of Endoscopes and Automated Endoscope Reprocessor
Australia										
AICE, 2019[13]	N/A		Manual ± AER[c]	N/A	AER required for HLD	Yes	Yes	Channel-purge cabinet required	No	Yes
GENCA/GESA, 2010[14]	N/A		Manual ± AER[c]	N/A	Either	Yes	Yes	Channel-purge or regular cabinet	No	Yes
Europe										
ESGE/ESGNA; Beilenhoff, 2017[15]	N/A		Manual ± AER[c]	Suggested	GI scopes HLD	Yes	Flush dry, no alcohol	Channel-purge or regular cabinet	No	Yes
French; Saviuc, 2015[16]	N/A		Manual ± AER	N/A	HLD for semicritical Sterilization for critical scopes	Yes	Flush dry, no alcohol[d]	Regular storage cabinet	No	Yes

British									
BSG, 2016[17]	N/A	Manual + AER[c]	N/A	AER required for HLD, sterilization for critical scopes	Yes	Flush dry, no alcohol	Channel purge recommended	No	Yes

Abbreviation: AICE, Australian Infection Control in Endoscopy; ASGE, American Society for Gastrointestinal Endoscopy; BSG, British Society of Gastroenterology; ESGE/ESGNA, European Society of Gastrointestinal Endoscopy/ European Society of Gastroenterology and Endoscopy Nurses and Associates; GENCA/GESA, Gastroenterological Nurses College of Australia/Gastroenterological Society of Australia; GI, Gastrointestinal; MEC, minimum effective concentration; N/A, not addressed; SGNA, Society of Gastroenterology Nurses and Associates.

a All the guidelines listed recommend that audits be done as part of a quality systems approach but often do not provide tools for such audits.

b ECRI 2019: safety alert warning against use of simethicone. Sites can opt to use simethicone based on clinical importance.

c Only AERs with validated cleaning cycles.

d All guidelines require monitoring of minimum effective concentration of liquid chemical HLD if it is a reusable formulation. All sterilization methods require biological indicators, chemical indicators, and review of cycle parameter printout to monitor various cycle parameters.

e Drying can be provided by manual flushing of air prior to storage or by AER with an air flush as part of the cycle.

Adapted from Alfa MJ, Singh HM. Impact of wet storage and other factors on biofilm formation and contamination of patient-ready endoscopes, a narrative review. Gastrointest Endosc 2020;91(2):236–47; with permission.

to the reprocessing area. The manual cleaning is crucial to ensure maximum removal of organic debris and microbes, thereby ensuring the efficacy of HLD or low-temperature sterilization. Ofstead and colleagues'[20] human factors study documented that only 1.5% of the 69 endoscopes evaluated had all 12 reprocessing steps completed and that only 43% had adequate manual cleaning. ANSI/AAMI ST91:2015[10] recommends monitoring of manual cleaning using rapid tests that assess organic or adenosine triphosphate (ATP) residuals. The rapid monitoring tests that have been utilized to evaluate cleaning of endoscope channels include tests for organic residues, such as protein, carbohydrate, hemoglobin, and tests for ATP.[21–28] Alfa and colleagues[21] reported that a busy endoscopy clinic was able to achieve a greater than 95% pass rate for adequate cleaning of endoscopes channels using a rapid ATP test whereas Visrodia and colleagues[26] reported only a 10% pass rate for manual cleaning of duodenoscopes. These studies indicate there is wide variation between endoscopy sites with respect to the current level of manual cleaning of endoscopes. The application of such rapid cleaning monitoring tests has been shown a valuable way to improve compliance of reprocessing personnel.[27,28] It was clear from Quan and colleagues'[27] study that ongoing monitoring of manual cleaning is important to ensure sustained compliance and to identify staff who persistently do not achieve the expected level of compliance. They reported that the most endoscope channel cleaning failures were attributed to staff who did not routinely reprocess endoscopes.[27] Ofstead and colleagues'[24] and Visrodia and colleagues'[25] studies clearly identified the extent of organic residuals reflecting inadequate cleaning using rapid organic test strips (eg, evaluate for protein, carbohydrate, and hemoglobin residuals) and rapid ATP testing. Despite the value of monitoring manual cleaning using rapid test for organic or ATP residuals, a recent survey by Thaker and colleagues[29] indicated that only 33.7% of 249 endoscopy clinics in the United States had implemented this recommendation.

The importance of using rapid tests to monitor manual cleaning is that endoscope channels found to have unacceptable levels of residuals can be recleaned prior to HLD or sterilization.[30] It is of little value to perform such rapid cleaning monitoring tests after the HLD or sterilization step because these processes fix any organic residuals to the surface, thereby making it harder to remove with the next round of cleaning.

Monitoring of manual cleaning using rapid tests for organic or ATP residuals should be done after the cleaning stage and NOT after HLD or sterilization.

There is a misconception that ATP monitoring after HLD or sterilization provides a rapid method to ensure there is no microbial contamination in patient-ready endoscopes. The concept that ATP levels are a rapid measure of microbial contamination in flexible endoscope channels has been shown to be incorrect because it takes between 10^2 colony-forming units (CFUs)/mL and 10^3 CFUs/mL to detect 1 relative light unit of bacterial ATP.[30] A recent study by McCafferty and colleagues[31] confirmed that ATP levels do not correlate with CFUs post-HLD. The current rapid ATP tests are not sensitive enough to ensure that there are not low levels of microbial contamination in patient-ready endoscopes. The core value of rapid ATP tests is to monitor cleaning efficacy after manual cleaning of flexible endoscopes.

Rapid ATP tests are appropriate for monitoring manual cleaning compliance but they CANNOT replace culture for detection of microbial contamination post-HLD or post-sterilization because they are not sensitive enough to detect low levels of viable organisms.

MONITORING DRY STORAGE

Ofstead and colleagues[32] and Thaker and colleagues[29] reported that only 45% and 7.8% of endoscopes, respectively, had forced air drying prior to storage. The extent of residual moisture in endoscope channels currently is not monitored and some guidelines indicate that the alcohol flush and air flush of an automated endoscope reprocessor (AER) cycle provide sufficient drying for storage.[9,10] Endoscopy reprocessing staff have a false sense of security that the AER alcohol flush and air flush cycle is sufficient to meet the manufacturer's instructions for use (MIFU) for dry storage—which is not true.[6]

Adequate drying to meet the endoscope MIFU for dry storage is NOT achieved by AER cycles that include an alcohol flush and air flush. This misconception leads to unrecognized wet storage of endoscope channels that promotes bacterial replication leading to biofilm or buildup biofilm.

Ofstead and colleagues'[24,32,33] and Barakat and colleagues'[34–36] utilization of thin borescopes to visualize the inside of endoscope channels of various inner diameters (eg, air, water, suction, and auxiliary channels) has provided an excellent tool that reprocessing staff can utilize to identify residuals after full reprocessing, such as organic debris, fluid, bristles, and so forth, as well as damage, such as perforations, channel folds, and so forth. **Fig. 1** shows the extent of moisture remaining after 24 hours to 48 hours storage in conventional storage cabinets of endoscopes that had been processed through an AER cycle that included an alcohol flush and forced air drying that was followed by an additional 10 minutes of manual forced air flushing.[33] **Fig. 2** shows growth detected from endoscope samples using the membrane filtration culture method.[33] It is clear that the AER cycle flushing combined with manual air flushing does not provide sufficient drying of endoscope channels to meet the MIFU for dry storage.[33–35] In addition, Ofstead and colleagues'[33] evaluation of Hydrion Humidicator Paper (Micro Essential Laboratory Inc., Brooklyn, NY) to monitor residual moisture during storage showed that it was an effective (95.5% positive predictive value and 100% negative predictive value compared with borescope assessment on the same endoscope) but less expensive alternative to the use of a borescopes. Ofstead and colleagues'[24,28,32,33,37] studies clearly identified the extent of organic residuals reflecting inadequate cleaning and the wet storage problem and further identified the role of simethicone in wet storage.

The inability to remove simethicone by current MIFU cleaning instructions and the impact of simethicone in preventing drying of endoscope channels have been confirmed by Barakat and colleagues'[34–36] studies. Simethicone has been used for years to reduce bubbles and froth that interfere with visualization of the gut mucosa. The impact that simethicone (or other off-label products used during clinical endoscopy procedures[37]), however, on reprocessing of endoscopes has not been considered in endoscope reprocessing guidelines (see **Table 1**). As outlined in a 2018 Emergency Care Research Institute alert,[38] the endoscope manufacturers have recommended against the use of non–water-soluble additives, such as simethicone, but indicate if sites felt it was clinically warranted it could be used. Subsequent position statements have been published supporting the value of simethicone in terms of polyp detection.[39–42] Further research is needed to clarify the role of simethicone residuals in drying of endoscope channels and whether or not these residuals promote biofilm or BBF formation that increases the risk of infection transmission.

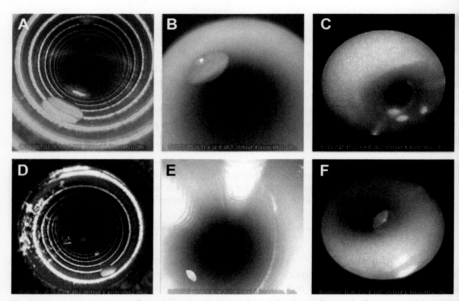

Fig. 1. Borescope image of residual moisture in an endoscope channel after overnight storage. Retained fluid droplets found inside endoscope channels. (*A*) Gastroscope, (*B*) colonoscope, (*C*) cystoscope, (*D*) gastroscope, (*E*) duodenoscope, and (*F*) Endoscopic ultrasound radial endoscope. (*From* Ofstead CL, Heymann OL, Quick MR, et al. Residual moisture and waterborne pathogens inside flexible endoscopes: Evidence from a multisite study of endoscope drying effectiveness. Am J Infect Control 2018; with permission.)

In terms of the impact of wet storage, Perumpail and colleagues'[43] study clearly documented that if endoscope channels contain moisture and low levels of *Pseudomonas aeruginosa* that multiple logs of replication can occur when the endoscope is stored overnight in a standard storage cabinet but not in a storage cabinet that purges air through the channels. As such, the reliance on the AER drying capability may partially contribute as a root cause to the unexpected level of high-concern organisms reported in the preliminary results of the FDA 522 postmarket clinical study.[2] In addition, the FDA[18] and Association for the Advancement of Medical Instrumentation (AAMI)[19] requirements of manufacturers to validate the cleaning efficacy of their endoscope reprocessing instructions do not require validation for removal of biofilm or buildup biofilm,[44] nor do they evaluate the impact of biofilm or buildup biofilm on the efficacy of HLD and sterilization.

Critical aspects of endoscope reprocessing that should be routinely monitored include adequacy of manual cleaning and residual moisture in channels after overnight storage.

ENDOSCOPE CULTURE MONITORING

Transmission of infections due to contaminated endoscopes is recognized as 1 of the top 10 patient safety issues.[45] Thaker and colleagues'[29] survey data from 249 endoscopy clinics in the United States indicated that only 53% of these clinics did periodic culture of their duodenoscopes. There are no published data (to the

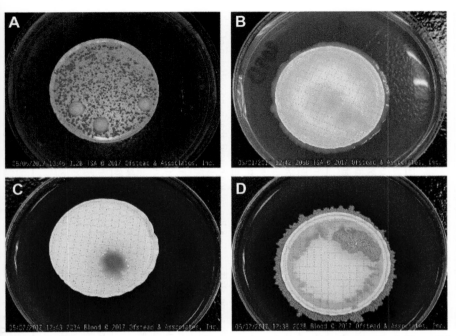

Fig. 2. .Photographs A,B,C,D represent culture results using the filtration method. (*From* Of-stead CL, Heymann OL, Quick MR, et al. Residual moisture and waterborne pathogens inside flexible endoscopes: Evidence from a multisite study of endoscope drying effectiveness. Am J Infect Control 2018; with permission.)

author's knowledge) on the extent of culture implementation for other types of en-doscopes in North America. Part of the hesitancy to perform culture has been the lack of a standardized culture protocol for endoscope channels. This has been addressed, however, as the FDA/Centers for Disease Control and Prevention (CDC)/American Society for Microbiology (ASM)[46] have released a validated sam-ple collection and culture protocol for duodenoscopes. This duodenoscope proto-col is only for samples collected from the biopsy port to the distal end, the elevator wire channel (for unsealed models), and the lever recess region. It is based on a flush-brush-flush sampling method and includes the addition of neutralizer and concentration of the sample by filtration (see **Fig. 2**) or centrifugation.[46] The 3 main endoscope manufacturers have validated that extraction efficacy is between 35% and 100%.[46] Endoscope sample collection kits are commercially available that provide all the materials to ensure compliance with the FDA/CDC/ASM[46] collection protocol. The recent August 29, 2019, FDA safety alert[3] has recommen-ded that endoscopy sites use this duodenoscope culture protocol to test their duo-denoscopes to better understand their site-specific contamination rates. They also have recommended that the contamination rates be provided to patients so they are aware of these prior to their duodenoscope procedure.

IMPLEMENTATION OF A QUALITY MANAGEMENT SYSTEM

The recent review by McCafferty and colleagues[47] indicated that the main factors contributing to infection transmission related to contaminated endoscopes include

Table 2
Overview of essential steps related to endoscope reprocessing

Essential Steps	Monitoring	Data Analysis and Action
Procedural (ie, aspects of patient procedures that affect reprocessing)	• Determine if lubricants, defoaming agents, tissue glue, etc. are used for any patient procedure. • Documentation of any endoscope problems (blockage, accessory extraction problems, broken accessories, etc.)	• Document facility approval for all off-label substances used. • Frequency of endoscope problems and documentation of response and corrective actions taken
Preclean	• Document completion for each scope; staff sign-off.	• Percentage missed, that is, no staff sign-off • Documentation of corrective actions taken.
Prolonged time in transit (eg, >1 h)	• Document time that preclean completed and time manual cleaning starts.	• Document percentage with prolonged transit. • Document that additional cleaning was performed when prolonged transit occurs. • If due to after-hours emergency procedures; develop after-hours reprocessing staff plan.
Leak test	• Document completion for each scope; staff sign-off	• Percentage missed, that is, no staff sign-of • Percentage leak test failure rate • Documentation of corrective actions taken
Manual clean	• Rapid testing of cleaning compliance; for example, ATP or organic residuals (minimally, testing of some scopes each day) • Document initial testing, recleaning and retest.	• Percentage failure rate • Percentage failure after reclean • Data review with reprocessing staff (weekly or monthly) • Individual data should be part of ongoing documentation of staff competency.
Visual inspection	• Document completion for each scope (define abnormalities to check: oily or other deposits, epoxy integrity, lens integrity, etc.); can use borescope for magnification during external visual inspection. • Staff sign-off	• Percentage missed, that is, no staff sign-off • Percentage faults detected • Document corrective actions taken. • Return rates to manufacturer

Disinfection/sterilization	• Test and document, minimum effective concentration of disinfectant, biological indicator, chemical indicator as appropriate; AER; document submicron filter changes. • Monthly culture of endoscope channels and/or final AER rinse water (if done at this endoscopy site)	• Percentage failures detected • AER; documentation of culture results and corrective actions taken if CFU exceeds limits (if done at this endoscopy site)
Drying/storage	• Document at least 10-min automated drying performed for each scope if external automated drying pump is used; staff sign-off. • Document function of drying pump (external flushing pump or channel-purge storage cabinet) as per MIFU. • Hydrion humidicator paper test or borescope test of scope channels after overnight storage (minimally test some scopes each week) • Internal channel inspection by borescope; monthly for each scope (define actionable lesions) • Culture of endoscope channels on periodic basis (if done at this endoscopy site)	• Percentage missed drying: that is, no staff sign-off • Percentage failure of drying based on hydrion humidicator paper test or borescope inspection • Percentage abnormalities identified by borescope inspection. Monthly summary of borescope abnormalities reviewed with reprocessing staff • Document corrective actions taken for any lapses detected in monitoring.
Documentation	• All monitoring records summarized and reviewed • Sign-off by supervisor	• Review all monitoring data and corrective actions taken with reprocessing staff on weekly basis and with infection control on monthly basis. • Include monitoring data in yearly competency review for each reprocessing staff person.

(continued on next page)

Table 2
(continued)

Essential Steps	Monitoring	Data Analysis and Action
Staff competency	• Initial training • Ongoing yearly competency	• Formal training related to endoscope reprocessing (for ALL types of endoscopes processed) with monitoring and supervisor sign-off on adequate demonstrated competency • Yearly competency review of all reprocessing personnel for all types of endoscopes processed. Supervisor sign-off of competency for each staff person for each type of endoscope processed.

Adapted from Alfa MJ, Singh HM. Impact of wet storage and other factors on biofilm formation and contamination of patient-ready endoscopes, a narrative review. GIE 2019 (accepted for publication Sept 2019); with permission.

lapses in reprocessing (eg, poor cleaning), inadequate drying, biofilm formation, endoscope design issues, and endoscope damage. Although a quality management system (QMS) cannot address endoscope design issues, QMS would be helpful in reducing the other main factors identified by McCafferty and colleagues.[47]

The American National Standards Institute (ANSI)/AAMI ST90 guideline[48] for QMS for reprocessing in health care is excellent but it does not address specific QMS issues related to endoscope reprocessing. Despite this limitation, it is a valuable document for establishing the overall approach to QMS in health care. The need for endoscopy clinics to review their practices has been highlighted by the CDC advisory in 2015.[49] This was furthered in 2016 when Provincial Infectious Diseases Advisory Committee (PIDAC)[7] advised: "If the health care facility has not recently conducted observational audits of endoscope reprocessing, and particularly duodenoscope reprocessing, it must conduct an audit immediately and then repeat audits regularly (annually at the minimum) or when practices change." Furthermore, the CDC have developed a user-friendly modifiable document specifically aimed at endoscope reprocessing.[50] This is an excellent document that sites can modify to reflect site-specific parameters.

> There is an urgent need to ensure implementation of a QMS that is specific to endoscope reprocessing.

There are some critical aspects, however, that are not reflected in the monitoring recommended by the CDC document.[50] The 2 critical stages in endoscope reprocessing that had the most errors were identified by Ofstead and colleagues'[20] human factor study and included manual cleaning and drying prior to storage. The importance of considering clinical changes that might affect cleaning and/or drying of endoscope channels (simethicone, tissue glue, and so forth) also has been established by Ofstead and colleagues.[37] All these published studies provide an impetus for establishing a QMS for monitoring critical aspects of endoscope reprocessing.

Table 2 outlines an overview of monitoring for various stages in endoscope reprocessing. Implementing this outline will provide data to indicate what the current compliance is with critical steps in endoscope reprocessing and will direct where improvements to endoscope reprocessing could be implemented.

SUMMARY

As stated by Thaker and colleagues,[29] it is "alarming" that there is such poor compliance with the multisociety guideline[11] that recommends thorough gastrointestinal endoscope drying prior to storage. Furthermore, there is an urgent need to introduce monitoring of critical stages in endoscope reprocessing so that the process is not hobbled by "we don't know what we don't know." Once endoscopy reprocessing sites have data from their QMS monitoring, they can implement changes to reduce the use of off-label products that cannot be effectively removed by MIFU cleaning, improve transit time between patient use and cleaning, optimize manual cleaning efficacy prior to HLD, ensure adequate drying for storage, and culture to reduce the risk of infection transmission due to contaminated endoscopes.

DISCLOSURE

M.J. Alfa has provided consulting services for 3M, Olympus, J&J, Healthmark, Novaflux, Ambu, and STERIS.

REFERENCES

1. FDA orders duodenoscope manufacturers to conduct postmarket surveillance studies in health care facilities. 2015. Available at: http://www.fda.gov/NewsEvents/Newsroom/PressAnnouncements/UCM465639. Accessed March 29, 2019.

2. FDA Statement; Statement from Jeff Shuren, MD, Director of the Center for Devices and Radiological Health, on continued efforts to assess duodenoscope contamination risk. 2019. Available at: https://www.accessdata.fda.gov/scripts/cdrh/cfdocs/cfPMA/pss.cfm. Accessed April 18, 2019.

3. The FDA is Recommending Transition to Duodenoscopes with Innovative Designs to Enhance Safety: FDA Safety Communication. 2019. Available at: https://www.fda.gov/medical-devices/safety-communications/fda-recommending-transition-duodenoscopes-innovative-designs-enhance-safety-fda-safety-communication. Accessed July 23, 2020.

4. ANSI/AAMI ST90:2017 Processing of health care products - Quality management systems for processing in health care facilities. Association for the Advancement of Medical Instrumentation (AAMI). Available at: www.aami.org. Accessed July 23, 2020.

5. ANSI/AAMI ST79:2010. Comprehensive guide to steam sterilization and sterility assurance in health care facilities. 2010 Association for the Advancement of Medical Instrumentation (AAMI). Available at: www.aami.org. Accessed July 23, 2020.

6. Alfa MJ, Singh HM. Impact of wet storage and other factors on biofilm formation and contamination of patient-ready endoscopes, a narrative review. Gastrointest Endosc 2020;91(2):236–47.

7. PIDAC Provincial Infectious Diseases Advisory Committee. Annex A—Minimizing the risk of bacterial transmission from patient to patient when using duodenoscopes. Annexed to: Best practices for cleaning, disinfection and sterilization of medical equipment/devices in all health care settings. Ontario Agency for Health Protection and Promotion (Public Health Ontario). Toronto (Ontario): Queen's Printer for Ontario; 2016. Accessed May 1, 2019.

8. Public Health Agency of Canada. Infection prevention and control guideline for flexible gastrointestinal endoscopy and flexible bronchoscopy. Ottawa, ON: Her Majesty the Queen in Right of Canada. 2010. Available at: www.phac-aspc.gc.ca/nois-sinp/guide/endo/pdf/endo-eng.pdf. Accessed March 26, 2019.

9. SGNA Standards of Infection Prevention in Reprocessing of Flexible Gastrointestinal Endoscopes 2016; Society of Gastroenterology Nurses and Associates, Inc (publisher). Available at: https://www.sgna.org/Practice-Resources/Infection-Prevention-old/Infection-Prevention-Toolkit/Professional-Society-Guidelines. Accessed March 29, 2019.

10. ANSI/AAMI ST91:2015 Flexible and semi-rigid endoscope processing in health care facilities. American National Standards Institute Inc, Association for the Advancement of Medical Instrumentation (publisher). ISBN 1-57020-585-X.

11. Reprocessing Guideline Task Force, Petersen BT, Cohen J, Hambrick RD III, et al. Multisociety guideline on reprocessing flexible GI endoscopes: 2016 update. Gastrointest Endosc 2017;85:282–94.e1.

12. Calderwood AH, Lukejohn WD, Muthusamy R, et al. Infection control during GI endoscopy. Quality Assurance Committee of the American Society for Gastrointestinal Endoscopy. Gastrointestinal Endoscopy; 2018. https://doi.org/10.1016/j.gie.2017.12.009.

3. Devereaux BM, Athan E, Brown RB, et al. Australian infection control in endoscopy consensus statements on carbapenemase-producing Enterobacteriaceae. J Gastroenterol Hepatol 2019 Apr;34(4):650–8.

4. GENCA/GESA/AGEA Infection Control in Endoscopy 2010. Gastroenterological Nurses College of Australia, Gastroenterological Society of Australia, Australia Gastrointestinal Endoscopy Society.

5. Beilenhoff U, Biering H, Blum R, et al. Prevention of multidrug-resistant infections from contaminated duodenoscopes: Position Statement of the European Society of Gastrointestinal Endoscopy (ESGE) and European Society of Gastroenterology Nurses and Associates (ESGENA). Endoscopy 2017;49:1098–106.

6. Saviuc P, Picot-Guéraud R, Sing JSC, et al. Evaluation of the quality of reprocessing of gastrointestinal endoscopes. Infect Control Hosp Epidemiol 2015. https://doi.org/10.1017/ice.2015.123.

7. British Society of Gastroenterology Guidance for decontamination of equipment for gastrointestinal endoscopy. Available at: https://www.bsg.org.uk/resource/guidance-on-decontamination-of-equipment-for-gastrointestinal-endoscopy-2017-edition.html. Accessed March 26, 2019.

8. Reprocessing medical devices in health care settings: validation methods and labeling guidance for industry and Food and drug administration staff. FDA Publisher; 2015. Available at: http://www.fda.gov/downloads/MedicalDevices/DeviceRegulationandGuidance/GuidanceDocuments/UCM080268.pdf. Accessed August 23, 2019.

9. AAMI TIR12:2010. Designing, testing, and labeling reusable medical devices for reprocessing in health care facilities: a guide for medical device manufacturers. Association for the Advancement of Medical Instrumentation (AAMI) Publishers; 2010. Available at: www.aami.org.

10. Ofstead CL, Wetzler HP, Snyder AK, et al. Endoscope reprocessing methods: A prospective study on the impact of human factors and automation. Gastroenterol Nurs 2010;33:304–11.

11. Alfa MJ, Fatima I, Olson N. The ATP test is a rapid and reliable audit tool to assess manual cleaning adequacy of flexible endoscope channels. Am J Infect Control 2013;41:249–53.

12. Alfa MJ N. Olson Simulated-use validation of a sponge ATP method for determining the adequacy of manual cleaning of endoscope channels. BMC Res Notes 2016;9:258.

13. Alfa MJ, Olson N, Degagne P, et al. Development and validation of rapid use scope test strips (RUST) to determine the efficacy of manual cleaning for flexible endoscope channels. Am J Infect Control 2012;40(9):860–5.

14. Ofstead CL, Wetzler HP, Heymann OL, et al. Longitudinal assessment of reprocessing effectiveness for colonoscopes and gastroscopes: Results of visual inspections, biochemical markers, and microbial cultures. Am J Infect Control 2017;45(2):e26–33.

15. Visrodia KH, Ofstead CL, Yellin HL, et al. The use of rapid indicators for the detection of organic residues on clinically used gastrointestinal endoscopes with and without visually apparent debris. Infect Control Hosp Epidemiol 2014;35(8):987–94.

16. Visrodia K, Hanada Y, Pennington KM, et al. Duodenoscope reprocessing surveillance with adenosine triphosphate testing and terminal cultures: A clinical pilot study. Gastrointest Endosc 2017;86(1):180–6.

27. Quan E, Mahmood R, Naik A, et al. Use of adesnosine triphosphate to audit re processing of flexible endoscopes with an elevator mechanism. Am J Infect Con trol 2018;46:1272–7.

28. Sethi S, Huang RJ, Barakat MT, et al. Adenosine triphosphate bioluminescence for bacteriologic surveillance and reprocessing strategies for minimizing risk o infection transmission by duodenoscopes. Gastrointest Endosc 2017;85 1180–7.e1.

29. Thaker AM, Muthusamy VR, Sedarat A, et al. Duodenoscope reprocessing prac tice patterns in U.S. endoscopy centers: a survey study. Gastrointest Endosc 2018;88:316–22.

30. Alfa MJ, Fatima I, Olson N. Validation of ATP to audit manual cleaning of flexible endoscope channels. Am J Infect Control 2011. https://doi.org/10.1016/j.ajic 2012.03.018.

31. McCafferty C,E, Abi-Hanna D, Aghajani MJ, et al. The validity of adenosine triphosphate (ATP) measurement in detecting endoscope contamination J Hosp Infect 2018. https://doi.org/10.1016/j.jhin.2018.08.004.

32. Ofstead CL, Wetzler HP, Johnson EA, et al. Simethicone residue remains inside gastrointestinal endoscopes despite reprocessing. Am J Infect Control 2016 https://doi.org/10.1016/j.ajic.2016.05.016.

33. Ofstead CL, Heymann OL, Quick MR, et al. Residual moisture and waterborne pathogens inside flexible endoscopes: Evidence from a multisite study of endo scope drying effectiveness. Am J Infect Control 2018. https://doi.org/10.1016/j ajic.2018.03.002.

34. Barakat MT, Girotra M, Huang RJ, et al. Scoping the scope: endoscopic evalua tion of endoscope working channels with a new high-resolution inspection endo scope (with video). Gastrointest Endosc 2018;88(4):601–11.e1.

35. Barakat MT, Huang RJ, Banerjee S. Comparison of automated and manual drying in the eliminating residual endoscope working channel fluid after reprocessing (with video). Gastrointest Endosc 2018. https://doi.org/10.1016/j.gie.2018 08.033.

36. Barakat MT, Huang RJ, Banerjee S. Simethicone is retained in endoscopes despite reprocessing: impact of its use on working channel fluid retention and adenosine triphosphate bioluminescence values (with video). Gastrointest En dosc 2018. https://doi.org/10.1016/j.gie.2018.08.012.

37. Ofstead CL, Hopkins KM, Eiland JE, et al. Widespread clinical use of simethi cone, insoluble lubricants, and tissue glue during endoscopy: A call to action for infection preventionists. Am J Infect Control 2019. https://doi.org/10.1016/j ajic.2019.02.0.

38. ECRI Alert A31187 : Olympus-Flexible Endoscopes: Manufacturer Recommends against Use of Simethicone/Non-Water Soluble Additives. 2018. Printed from Health Devices Alerts on Friday, Available at: www.ecri.org. Accessed March 19, 2019.

39. Kutyla M, O'Connor S, Gurusamy S, et al. Influence of simethicone added to the rinse water during colonoscopies on polyp detection rates: results of an unin tended cohort study. Digestion 2018;98:217–21.

40. Monrroy H, Vargas JI, Glasinovic E, et al. Use of N-acetylcysteine plus simethi cone to improve mucosal visibility during upper GI endoscopy: a double blind randomized, controlled study. Gastrointest Endosc 2018;87:986–93.

41. Liu X, Guan CT, He S, et al. Effect of premedication on lesion detection rate and visualization of the mucosa during upper gastrointestinal endoscopy: a

multicenter large sample randomized controlled double-blind study. Surg Endosc 2018;88:3548–56.

42. Benmassaoud A, Parent J. CAG position statement: canadian association of gastroenterology position statement on the impact of simethicone on endoscope reprocessing. J Can Assoc Gastroenterol 2018;1:40–2. Accessed March 25, 2019.

43. Perumpail RB, Marya NB, McGinty BL, et al. Endoscope reprocessing: Comparison of drying effectiveness and microbial levels with an automated drying and storage cabinet with forced filtered air and a standard storage cabinet. Am J Infect Control 2019. https://doi.org/10.1016/j.ajic/2019.02.016.

44. Alfa MJ, Ribeiro MM, da Costa Luciano C, et al. A novel polytetrafluoroethylene-channel model, which simulates low levels of culturable bacteria in buildup biofilm after repeated endoscope reprocessing. Gastrointest Endosc 2017;86: 442–51.

45. ECRI Institute. Executive Brief: top 10 health technology hazards for 2018. Plymouth Meeting (PA): ECRI Institute; 2017. p. 5.

46. Duodenoscope surveillance sampling & culturing; reducing the risks of infection. Food and Drug Administration, Centers for Disease Control, American Society for Microbiology; 2018.

47. McCafferty CE, Aghajani MJ, Abi-Hanna D, et al. An update on gastrointestinal endoscopy-associated infections and their contributing factors. Ann Clin Microbiol Antimicrob 2018;17:36.

48. ANSI/AAMI ST90:2017. Processing of health care products—Quality management systems for processing in health care facilities. Association for the Advancement of Medical Instrumentation (publisher). ISBN 978-1-57020-676-4.

49. Center for Disease Control Advisory. Immediate Need to Review Procedures for Cleaning, Disinfecting and Sterilizing Reusable Devices. Infection Control Today 2015. Available at: https://www.infectioncontroltoday.com/sterile-processing/immediate-need-review-procedures-cleaning-disinfecting-and-sterilizing-reusable. Accessed August 20, 2019.

50. Centre for Disease Control essential Elements of a reprocessing program for flexible endoscopes – recommendations of the HICPAC. 2017. Available at: https://www.cdc.gov/hicpac/recommendations/flexible-endoscope-reprocessing.html. Accessed April 12, 2019.

Recent Actions by the US Food and Drug Administration

Reducing the Risk of Infection from Reprocessed Duodenoscopes

Shanil P. Haugen, PhD*, Ann Ferriter, Jian Connell, DNP, MSN, CPN,
Lauren J. Min, PhD, Hanniebey D. Wiyor, PhD, RAC,
Stephanie Cole, PhD

KEYWORDS

• FDA • Reprocessing • Duodenoscopes • Infection

KEY POINTS

- US Food and Drug Administration staff outline recent actions undertaken to reduce the risk of infection from reprocessed duodenoscopes.
- Actions such as device design changes and improved reprocessing instructions have improved the safety of these devices, but additional work is needed.
- Looking forward, engagement and collaboration among the wider community of stakeholders will be beneficial toward reducing the risk of infection from reprocessed duodenoscopes. Such a community can address unanswered questions that merit further research and develop tools that can be used by health care facilities to improve the quality of reprocessing at their sites.

INTRODUCTION

The Food and Drug Administration (FDA) is the oldest comprehensive consumer protection agency in the United States. The FDA oversight of food and drugs began in 1906. Since then, Congress has expanded the FDA's role in protecting and promoting the development of human and veterinary drugs, biological products, medical devices and radiation-emitting products, human and animal food, cosmetics, and tobacco. Congress responded to the public's desire for more oversight over medical devices by passing the Medical Device Amendments to the Federal Food, Drug, and Cosmetic

United States Food and Drug Administration, Office of Medical Products and Tobacco, Center for Devices and Radiological Health, Office of Health Technology 3, 10903 New Hampshire Avenue, Silver Spring, MD 20993-0002, USA
* Corresponding author.
E-mail address: Shanil.Haugen@fda.hhs.gov

Gastrointest Endoscopy Clin N Am 30 (2020) 711–721
https://doi.org/10.1016/j.giec.2020.06.010
1052-5157/20/Published by Elsevier Inc.
giendo.theclinics.com

Act in 1976, and subsequent updates, including the 21st Century Cures Act. The FDA monitors the ongoing safety and effectiveness of regulated marketed medical devices and that includes endoscopes used in gastroenterology procedures.

Endoscopic retrograde cholangiopancreatography (ERCP) procedures combine upper gastrointestinal (GI) endoscopy with fluoroscopic imaging to evaluate—as well as treat—conditions involving the biliary tree and pancreas with a specialized endoscope called a duodenoscope. The unique design of duodenoscopes enables clinicians to perform ERCP procedures. Duodenoscopes have more complex features than other endoscopes, however, which can present significant challenges for reprocessing them in preparation for safe use in subsequent patients. Duodenoscopes contain many small working parts with difficult-to-reach crevices. Therefore, if a duodenoscope is not meticulously cleaned and reprocessed, living microbes harboring in residual tissue or fluid from a prior procedure can be transmitted via the scope to a subsequent patient. In rare cases, this can lead to patient-to-patient transmission of infection.

In the fall of 2013, the Centers for Disease Control and Prevention (CDC) alerted the FDA to a potential association of multidrug-resistant bacteria and duodenoscopes. Since that time, FDA has taken several actions to reduce the risk of infection associated with these life-saving devices. Regulation of these devices, currently available data, and a timeline of FDA's actions are summarized in this article. This article closes by discussing the future of duodenoscope design and use.

PREMARKET EVALUATION OF DUODENOSCOPES

Duodenoscopes are Class II medical devices regulated under 21 Code of Federal Regulations 876.1500, Endoscopes and accessories.[1] Under these regulations, duodenoscope manufacturers must submit 510(k) premarket notifications to the FDA prior to marketing new duodenoscopes in the United States. Duodenoscopes used for ERCP have been in use in the United States prior to the initiation of FDA's regulation of medical devices in 1976. Throughout the ensuing decades, manufacturers have made modifications to duodenoscopes, including but not limited to improved optics, handling, reprocessing methods, material changes, and other design changes. Manufacturers are required to submit to FDA a new 510(k) application for a device modification if the change could affect the safety or effectiveness of the device.

Currently, the FDA's premarket evaluation of duodenoscopes often includes evaluation of the following performance tests or assessments:

- Electrical safety
- Thermal safety
- Electromagnetic compatibility
- Optical performance tests
- Functionality tests
- Mechanical tests
- Biocompatibility
- Reprocessing validation
- Human factors
- Postmarket adverse event and recall reporting information

Prior to 2015, in accordance with the then-current FDA guidance document, "Labeling Reusable Medical Devices for Reprocessing in Health Care Facilities: FDA Reviewer Guidance," dated April 1996, 510(k) premarket submissions included statements attesting to FDA that the device manufacturer had or would complete reprocessing validation to support their reprocessing instructions for use. Section 3059 of the 21st Century Cures Act of 2016 (Public Law 114–255) required the FDA to publish a list of reusable medical devices for which validated reprocessing instructions and the validation data for reprocessing of the reusable device must be included in a 510(k) submission. This section of the Act also gives FDA the authority to render a 510(k) decision that these reusable devices are not substantially equivalent to a predicate device, if the validated instructions for use and reprocessing validation data submitted as part of the 510(k) are inadequate. Duodenoscopes were included in the list of reusable medical devices published in the *Federal Register* on June 9, 2017 (82 FR 26807).[2]

Duodenoscope manufacturers typically include in 510(k) submissions durability testing to assess the impact of multiple simulated clinical and reprocessing uses on the functionality of the device; however, the test methodology varies among different duodenoscope manufacturers.

DUODENOSCOPE DESIGN

Most duodenoscope models marketed in the United States are reusable medical devices and require the user to process (ie, clean and high-level disinfect [HLD] or sterilize) the device for initial use as well as reprocess the device after each use.

The availability of different duodenoscope models and designs in the United States is changing. In the past few years, some duodenoscope models were withdrawn from the market, while at the same time new duodenoscope models have gained marketing clearance.

Design Aspects of Duodenoscopes Marketed in the United States

The duodenoscope has a complex device design, which presents a particular challenge to cleaning, HLD, and sterilization. Duodenoscopes are more complex than most other endoscopes, such as gastroscopes or colonoscopes, in that the device contains a working channel that comes off the side of the scope to allow cannulation of the bile duct under direct visualization. Unlike most other endoscopes, duodenoscopes have a movable elevator mechanism at the tip. Raising the elevator mechanism changes the angle of the accessory instrument exiting the instrument channel, allowing the instrument to access and treat problems with fluid drainage from the bile ducts or pancreas. The FDA's engineering assessment and literature review, however, have identified the elevator mechanism as a feature that makes reprocessing of duodenoscopes challenging.[3] For example, 1 step of the manual cleaning instructions in the device's labeling is to brush the elevator area. The moving parts of the elevator mechanism introduce microscopic crevices that may not be reached with a brush. Failure to remove all body fluids and organic debris may result in persistent microbial contamination of the device. Microbes may survive in residual body fluids and organic debris despite immersion of the duodenoscope in HLD solution, potentially exposing subsequent patients to infectious organisms.

Elevator Wire Channel

Duodenoscopes have a long thin wire that connects the elevator control mechanism (on the control handle) to the elevator at the distal tip of the endoscope (the end inserted into the patient). That wire is housed in a narrow channel called the elevator wire channel, which spans from the distal tip to the control handle. Manipulating the elevator control on the control handle moves the elevator wire and subsequently moves the elevator mechanism at the distal end of the scope. In some models of duodenoscopes, the elevator wire channel is open or unsealed allowing patient body fluids or organic debris to enter the elevator wire channel. That open elevator wire channel requires reprocessing by flushing detergent into the channel for cleaning, followed by the flushing of HLD into the channel for HLD. Newer designs with closed or sealed elevator wire channels eliminate the requirement to reprocess the elevator wire channel.

Currently, only the Olympus TJF-160VF/F, the Olympus JF-140F, and the Olympus PJF-160 have open elevator wire channels. As discussed later, the remaining reusable duodenoscope models have a closed or sealed-off elevator wire channel, which is intended to prevent soil from entering this channel.

The FDA worked closely with all 3 manufacturers of reusable duodenoscopes in the United States (Fujifilm, Olympus, and Pentax) as they evaluated the sealing mechanisms for the elevator wire channels in their duodenoscopes. All 3 manufacturers made design changes to provide an additional margin of safety in an effort to reduce the risk of fluid ingress and cross-contamination. After FDA clearance of these devices with the design changes, these companies conducted recalls to bring the duodenoscopes up to the new specifications: Olympus TJF-Q180V (K143153, cleared in January 2016), Fujifilm ED-530XT (K152257, cleared in July 2017), and Pentax ED-3490TK (K161222 cleared in February 2018; previously cleared in K092710).

All new reusable duodenoscope models with sealed elevator wire channels are expected to undergo robust performance testing to demonstrate adequate sealing, which is important to ensure that the design requirement is met (21 Code of Federal Regulations 820.30).

Accessibility to Crevices at the Distal End

As discussed at the May 2015 panel meeting, the FDA engineering assessment revealed similarities among the 3 reusable duodenoscopes manufacturers' designs for sealing off the elevator wire channel. Very small crevices in the elevator recess and features, such as the O-ring, were exposed to patient soil. It is important to thoroughly clean these areas of the device to remove soil prior to subsequent processing of the device. A recent design change was implemented to improve accessibility to these crevices.

In addition, duodenoscopes are available with either fixed or removable distal caps. Distal caps are made of plastic, rubber, silicone, or other soft materials to cover the metal edges on duodenoscope distal ends to prevent tissue injury from the metal edges. Fixed endcap duodenoscopes have the cap permanently glued to the metal edges around the distal end, whereas removable distal caps remain on the duodenoscope by tension/friction.

During reprocessing, removable distal caps allow greater access to the elevator, including the underside of the elevator. This removable distal cap design is expected to improve the ability to clean the elevator recess and thus improve the safety of these devices.

Duodenoscopes with removable caps also eliminate the need for adhesive under the cap. As noted in FDA January 2017 Safety Communication,[4] cracks and gaps in the adhesive that seals the fixed distal caps can occur over time with repeat use. These cracks or gaps can lead to microbial and fluid ingress. These areas can be challenging to clean and HLD and may increase the risk of infection transmission among patients.

OOD AND DRUG ADMINISTRATION TIMELINE OF INVESTIGATIONS INTO UTBREAKS AND ACTIONS

ome of the activities in the FDA's investigation of duodenoscope-associated infec-
ons are summarized. This is not intended to be a comprehensive list of FDA activities
r actions, but rather a general overview.

all 2013–Winter 2014

he CDC alerted the FDA to a potential association between patients experiencing
ultidrug-resistant bacteria infections after ERCP procedures with duodenoscopes.
pon further investigation, the FDA learned that these new cases of infection were
ccurring despite confirmation that the users were following proper manufacturer
leaning and disinfection or sterilization instructions. The FDA communicated with
deral partners, manufacturers, and other stakeholders to better understand the crit-
al factors contributing to these infections and how to best mitigate them.

The FDA began reviewing the 510(k) history of all duodenoscope manufacturers and
ompleted an analysis of the adverse events submitted to FDA to identify trends asso-
iated with the duodenoscopes identified. An effort also was conducted to identify all
LD manufacturers and review the data to ensure that biofilm formation was not an
sue. The FDA began working with the CDC and US Environmental Protection Agency
EPA) to develop testing methods and a protocol to analyze different HLDs; this project
oncluded in 2014.

oring–Fall 2014

equests for information (RFIs) were distributed to the duodenoscope manufacturers
nd responses were received and reviewed. The FDA worked interactively with duo-
enoscope manufacturers, reviewing their validation study protocols and analyzing
ata from their cleaning HLD studies and recommending more rigorous testing with
ore robust cleaning and HLD protocols to enhance the safety margin associated
ith duodenoscopes use. The FDA repeatedly interacted with manufacturers to iden-
fy design features that may have contributed to the transmission of infection. The
DA also conducted a survey of a collaborative network of clinical sites to assess duo-
enoscope use and gathered information from hospitals regarding the use of HLDs
sed for reprocessing compared with sterilization capabilities with ethylene oxide.
uodenoscope surveillance culturing was discussed at the CDC Healthcare Infection
ontrol Practices Advisory Committee public meeting. Collaborative evaluation with
e EPA to assess effectiveness of HLDs was conducted.

Vinter–Spring 2015

he FDA conducted an evaluation of automated endoscope reprocessors (AERs),
cluding interactive review of manufacturer validation study protocols, analysis of
ata from cleaning and HLD or liquid chemical sterilization studies, and recommenda-
on for additional, more rigorous testing with more robust reprocessing protocols to
nhance the safety margin associated with duodenoscopes. Additional Medical Prod-
ct Safety Network interviews with hospital facilities that experienced clusters or out-
reaks of antibiotic-resistant bacterial infections related to ERCP procedures were
erformed.

May 2015 and Subsequent Actions

May 2015, the Gastroenterology and Urology Devices Panel met to discuss the re-
orted outbreaks of infections associated with the use of duodenoscopes during

ERCP procedures.[5] A summary of panel recommendations and FDA's subsequent activities is provided.

- The panel unanimously agreed that ERCP is an important procedure, and the benefits of ERCP outweigh the risk associated with the use of duodenoscope in appropriately selected patients; however, the panel found that duodeno scopes and AERs did not provide an acceptable level of effectiveness and safety During the panel meeting, there was a proposal to move toward sterilization rather than HLD of duodenoscopes, but sterilization was not unanimously recommended.
  ○ FDA action
     To address questions regarding the safety and effectiveness of current du odenoscope reprocessing practices, in October 2015, the FDA ordered the 3 duodenoscope manufacturers to conduct 2 postmarket surveillance studies: a human factors validation study for the reprocessing instruction and a microbiological sampling and culturing study. The FDA tracked progress and results from those studies and in March of 2018, the FDA is sued warning letters to the duodenoscope manufacturers for failing to comply with the postmarket surveillance study.
- The panel agreed that manual cleaning, in particular the brushing of channels and elevators, is a critical step in reprocessing duodenoscopes to ensure the removal of debris and subsequent proper disinfection or sterilization. Furthermore, to ensure manual cleaning is conducted properly and that users can follow the numerous complex steps, the panel recommended additional training for reproc essing personnel at health care facilities and the incorporation of human factor testing to evaluate reprocessing instructions.
  ○ FDA action
     In accordance with panel recommendations, the FDA requested that the manufacturers provide updated and newly validated duodenoscope re processing instructions that included an emphasis on effective cleaning of the elevator recess and additional brushing and flushing steps.
- The panel agreed that human factors testing for reprocessing instructions wa important to ensure reprocessing personnel will comprehend and correctl follow reprocessing instructions in the labeling.
  ○ FDA action
     As recommended by the panel, all reusable duodenoscopes that have sub sequently been cleared by FDA have included human factors validation testing of duodenoscope reprocessing instructions in the premarket sub mission, or human factors testing was ordered in postmarket studies.
- The panel discussed the CDC 2015 interim guidelines on surveillance fo contamination of duodenoscopes after reprocessing. The panel concluded that more data and validation testing was needed before a surveillance program should be implemented by health care facilities.
  ○ FDA action
     To address concerns about the lack of validation for sampling and culturing methods, the FDA worked with the CDC, the American Society for Micro biology, and other experts to develop a protocol for surveillance sampling and culturing of duodenoscopes. This protocol, which was used by duo denoscope manufacturers as part of their postmarket surveillance studies, was released publicly in February 2018 (https://www.fda.gov media/111081/download).

- The panel identified the need for development and validation of cleaning verification assays.
  - FDA action
    - To address the lack of validation and FDA clearance for cleaning verification assays, the FDA contacted manufacturers of adenosine triphosphate test systems advising them of the importance for manufacturing, testing, and labeling for medical devices promoted for assessing duodenoscope cleaning.
- The panel discussed informed consent and patient selection and recommended disclosure of the risks and alternatives to ERCP.
  - FDA action
    - In line with the panel's recommendations for transparency on the risks of ERCP, the FDA requested that duodenoscope manufacturers include in the revised device labeling the observed contamination rates from the postmarket studies.
- The panel recommended that manufacturers should be encouraged to redesign duodenoscopes to allow for thorough cleaning, disinfection, and sterilization.
  - FDA action
    - In line with the panel's recommendation for duodenoscope designs that allow for thorough reprocessing, the FDA requested changes to duodenoscope design to reduce the risk of ingress of fluids in sealed-off areas of the device. The FDA also requested that duodenoscope labeling be revised and include recommendations for annual inspection to identify and replace worn and damaged parts. The FDA subsequently has cleared duodenoscopes with disposable endcaps, which allow greater access for cleaning the elevator as well as a fully disposable duodenoscope, both of which are expected to have improved safety profiles relative to fixed end-cap duodenoscopes.
- The panel urged the FDA to provide early communication of the facts to the public in situations when the FDA has a medical device concern but not enough information to determine the most appropriate action toward a resolution.
  - FDA action
    - As recommended by the panel, the FDA issued multiple public communications to disclose currently available data. For example, following the panel meeting, the FDA issued an August 2015 communication of supplemental measures to enhance duodenoscope reprocessing that emerged from the May 2015 panel meeting. These optional supplemental measures that may be implemented by health care facilities include double HLD, sampling and culturing of duodenoscopes, ethylene oxide sterilization, and liquid chemical sterilization. The FDA also publicly communicated on the interim postmarket surveillance study data, which are discussed in more detail later.

In addition to the activities recommended by the panel, the FDA has continued regulatory oversight. The FDA has conducted directed inspections of the 3 US duodenoscope manufacturers, and, after the inspections, the FDA has issued warning letters for regulatory violations, when appropriate.

NOVEMBER 2019 PANEL MEETING

In November 2019, the General Hospital and Personal Use Devices Panel met to discuss the current infection, contamination, and postmarket duodenoscope data as well as current technological design advancements that potentially could enhance the safety of these devices.[6] The FDA relayed concerns that current practices for reprocessing duodenoscopes are not sufficient to avoid infections associated with ERCP. The following information was presented:

- Adverse event reports that were submitted to FDA indicate a decrease in the number of reported infections, with a concurrent increase in reports of contaminated duodenoscopes. The decrease in infections suggests that efforts to reduce the risk of infection from duodenoscopes have yielded improvements; however, additional improvements will be important to decrease the risk of infection further. Sampling and culturing of duodenoscopes after reprocessing were identified as supplemental measures to enhance duodenoscope reprocessing at the 2015 FDA panel meeting; the marked increase in reports of contamination may be due to the increasing number of facilities conducting duodenoscope sampling and culturing since 2015.
- Results from the FDA-mandated postmarket surveillance studies conducted by duodenoscope manufacturers showed that up to 6% of reprocessed duodenoscopes were contaminated with high-concern organisms (organisms that are associated more often with infections). The percent of contaminated samples shows that improvements are necessary to better assure patient safety. Initial root cause analyses suggest that some factors that may contribute to device contamination after reprocessing include device damage and errors in reprocessing; however, additional data are needed.
- Results of human factors validation testing of the reprocessing instructions indicated that current reprocessing user materials are difficult for reprocessing staff to read, understand, and follow. Study participants experienced difficulties and multiple failures in achieving adequate reprocessing tasks. Therefore, current reprocessing user materials do not adequately support user understanding and adherence to reprocessing instructions.

The panel was asked to comment on FDA's previous actions and whether the trajectory that FDA had taken to reduce the risk of infections continued to be appropriate. The consensus of the panel was that training of reprocessing personnel was of utmost importance. The panel recognized that such training falls outside of FDA's purview; nonetheless, FDA was encouraged to collaborate with manufacturers, accrediting organizations, and other stakeholders to ensure correct reprocessing of duodenoscopes in health care settings. Some panel members commented that the magnitude of the problem did not raise concerns and that FDA mandates on strategies to reduce the risk of infection for duodenoscopes would not be helpful. The panel recommended that the FDA carefully consider next steps and make deliberate decisions.

The FDA discussed standardizing duodenoscope durability testing that is conducted by the manufacturer. The panel's consensus was that standardized durability testing was appropriate, because damage to the duodenoscopes often was not recognized by health care personnel. The panel noted that the details of the durability testing should be further discussed and refined with industry.

The panel discussed the potential of new designs to reduce duodenoscope contamination rates and the urgency with which the transition should be made. The panel's consensus was that although new device designs have the potential to reduce contamination, at that time there were insufficient data to demonstrate that reduction. The panel commented that additional modifications to the device design and reprocessing instructions, education, and practices could be made.

The panel was asked to comment on the appropriate balance between obtaining ata premarket versus postmarket for assessing devices that are intended to reduce ne risk of infection from duodenoscopes. The panel noted that new device designs eed to demonstrate effectiveness in reducing the risk of contamination prior to being vailable for use; however, the panel recognized the challenges associated with enerating such data prior to marketing.

The panel discussed the adequacy/margin of safety for HLD as well as the chal-nges and benefits of sterilization for routine duodenoscope reprocessing. The anel's consensus was that cleaning is the most important step in duodenoscope eprocessing. The panel noted that in properly cleaned duodenoscopes, HLD is opropriate; however, panel members acknowledged that reports indicate that duo-enoscopes are not cleaned properly. The panel also discussed the challenges of nplementing sterilization of duodenoscopes, such as potential decreased patient ac-ess to ERCPs and increased costs.

JTURE DIRECTIONS

uodenoscopes serve a critical, and sometimes life-saving, function in evaluation and eatment of patients with biliary and certain pancreatic diseases. The FDA believes ne benefits of the availability of duodenoscopes to perform the ERCP procedure utweigh the risks in appropriately selected patients. The decreased number of re-orted infections since 2015 is encouraging and indicates that the efforts to reduce ne risks of infections have had success; however, the FDA continues to receive re-orts of infections, which means there is a continued need to improve the safety of eprocessed duodenoscopes. The FDA seeks to further improve the safety of ERCP y addressing the challenges associated with duodenoscope reprocessing due to s complex design and reprocessing challenges.

Several strategies have already been implemented to reduce the risk of duodeno-cope contamination, including

- Validated revisions to reprocessing instructions to include rigorous cleaning of the elevator recess
- Design changes to reduce the risk of inadvertent fluid ingress into the duodeno-scope and clearance of duodenoscopes with disposable components
- Collection of postmarket surveillance data to assess the effectiveness of current reprocessing practices on devices in use and new device designs
- Human factors evaluation of reprocessing instructions
- Development of a validated protocol for duodenoscope sampling and culturing
- Public communications to disclose currently available data
- Compliance activities, such as inspections and warning letters, to ensure duode-noscope design and manufacturing are in accordance with US quality systems requirements

Some activities are ongoing:

- Ensuring that cleaning verification assays have been appropriately validated
- Requesting transparency in labeling by including the observed contamination rate
- Publicly communicating on the need to transition to newer models of duodeno-scopes that simplify or eliminate cleaning

The FDA believes the best solution to reducing the risk of disease transmission by uodenoscopes is through innovative device designs that make reprocessing easier, more effective, or unnecessary. As stated in the August 2019 Safety Communication, the FDA now is recommending that hospitals and endoscopy facilities transition away from fixed endcap duodenoscopes to those with newer design features that facilitate or eliminate the need for reprocessing. The FDA recommends health care facilities consider making the transition to those devices when they become available. To verify that the new designs reduce the contamination rate, the FDA also has ordered the manufacturers of reusable duodenoscopes with disposable endcaps to conduct new postmarket surveillance studies. Upon completion of these postmarket surveillance studies, the FDA expects the labeling to be updated with contamination rate data.

The FDA recognizes that a transition away from conventional duodenoscopes to the newer, innovative models will take time due to cost and market availability. Health care facilities looking to make a transition to newer designs of devices may have questions about demonstrated benefits to those newer devices. The FDA encourages health care facilities purchasing new duodenoscopes to begin developing a transition plan and work to replace their conventional duodenoscopes with newer models.

In addition to technological advancements, engagement and collaboration among the wider community of stakeholders also will be beneficial toward reducing the risk of infection from reprocessed duodenoscopes. Such a community can raise awareness of the importance of duodenoscope cleaning, work to improve reprocessing training, identify the most pressing unanswered questions that merit further research, and also develop tools that can be used by health care facilities to improve the quality of reprocessing at their sites. The FDA looks forward to working with the community to further reduce the risk of infections from reprocessed duodenoscopes.

REFERENCES

1. U.S. Code of Federal Regulations Title 21, 876.1500 Endoscopes and accessories. Available at: https://www.accessdata.fda.gov/scripts/cdrh/cfdocs/cfcfr/cfrsearch.cfm?fr=876.1500. Accessed May 8, 2020.
2. U.S. Federal Register Notice, Volume 82, No. 110. Available at: https://www.govinfo.gov/content/pkg/FR-2017-06-09/pdf/2017-12007.pdf. Accessed May 8, 2020.
3. U.S. Food and Drug Administration. FDA Executive Summary Prepared for the May 14-15, 2015 meeting of the Gastroenterology-Urology Devices Panel of the Medical Devices Advisory Committee. Available at: https://wayback.archive-it.org/7993/20170113091323/http://www.fda.gov/downloads/AdvisoryCommittees/CommitteesMeetingMaterials/MedicalDevices/MedicalDevicesAdvisoryCommittee/Gastroenterology-UrologyDevicesPanel/UCM445592.pdf. Accessed May 8, 2020
4. U.S. FDA Safety Communication. Available at: https://www.fda.gov/medical devices/safety-communications/update-importance-following-validated-reprocessing-instructions-pentax-ed-3490tk-video-duodenoscopes. Accessed May 8, 2020.
5. U.S. Food and Drug Administration. 2015 Materials of the Gastroenterology-Urology Devices Panel. Available at: https://wayback.archive-it.org/7993/20170112002249/http:/www.fda.gov/AdvisoryCommittees/CommitteesMeetingMaterials/MedicalDevices/MedicalDevicesAdvisoryCommittee/Gastroenterology-UrologyDevicesPanel/ucm445590.htm. Accessed May 8, 2020.
6. U.S. Food and Drug Administration. November 6-7, 2019: General Hospital and Personal Use Devices Panel of the Medical Devices Advisory Committee Meeting Announcement. Available at: https://www.fda.gov/advisory committees/advisory-committee-calendar/november-6-7-2019-general-hospital

and-personal-use-devices-panel-medical-devices-advisory-committee#event-materials. Accessed May 8, 2020.
7. U.S. Food and Drug Administration. The FDA is Recommending Transition to Duodenoscopes with Innovative Designs to Enhance Safety: FDA Safety Communication. Available at: https://www.fda.gov/medical-devices/safety-communications/fda-recommending-transition-duodenoscopes-innovative-designs-enhance-safety-fda-safety-communication. Accessed May 8, 2020.

The Centers for Disease Control and Prevention Guidance on Flexible Gastrointestinal Endoscopes

Lessons Learned from Outbreaks, Infection Control

Isaac Benowitz, MD*, Heather A. Moulton-Meissner, PhD,
Lauren Epstein, MD, Matthew J. Arduino, DrPH

KEYWORDS

- Endoscope • Gastrointestinal • Duodenoscope • Outbreak • Infection
- Transmission • Disinfection • Cleaning

KEY POINTS

- Gastrointestinal flexible endoscopes are essential diagnostic and therapeutic instruments that also carry risks of transmitting pathogens to patients related to problems with device design or damage and inadequate adherence to reprocessing instructions.
- These devices should be cleaned and high-level disinfected after each patient use, or cleaned and sterilized after each patient use if there is an available sterilization method, according to the manufacturer's instructions for use.
- Possible endoscope-related transmission events and outbreaks and instances of failure to adhere to recommended reprocessing practices should be reported promptly to public health authorities; investigations can help identify opportunities to improve device design, use, and reprocessing.
- CDC Guideline for Disinfection and Sterilization in Healthcare Facilities, the Essential Elements of a Reprocessing Program for Flexible Endoscopes – The Recommendations of the Healthcare Infection Control Practices Advisory Committee (HICPAC), and the FDA/CDC/American Society for Microbiology Duodenoscope Surveillance Sampling & Culturing Protocols are free resources that contain guidance on flexible endoscope reprocessing, minimal expectations for a reprocessing program, and sampling and culturing of duodenoscopes and other endoscopes.

Division of Healthcare Quality Promotion, Centers for Disease Control and Prevention, 1600 Clifton Road Northeast, MS H16-3, Atlanta, GA 30329, USA
* Corresponding author.
E-mail address: ibenowitz@cdc.gov

Gastrointest Endoscopy Clin N Am 30 (2020) 723–733
https://doi.org/10.1016/j.giec.2020.06.009
1052-5157/20/Published by Elsevier Inc.

giendo.theclinics.com

INTRODUCTION

The Centers for Disease Control and Prevention (CDC) is the nation's health protec tion agency. The mission of the CDC Division of Healthcare Quality Promotion (DHQP) is to protect patients; protect health care personnel; and promote safety quality, and value in national and international health care delivery systems. DHQP develops infection control guidelines and resources with input from the Healthcare Infection Control Practices Advisory Committee (HICPAC), a federal advisory com mittee appointed to provide advice and guidance to the Department of Health and Human Services and to CDC regarding the practice of infection control and strate gies for surveillance, prevention, and control of health care–associated infections antimicrobial resistance, and related events in US health care settings. DHQP assist with investigation and response to emerging health care–associated threat: including those resulting in adverse events among patients and health car personnel. The DHQP also works with public and private partners to prevent the spread of antimicrobial resistance.

Flexible endoscopes are diagnostic and therapeutic instruments used to visualize the interior of hollow organs and collect tissue samples. Gastrointestinal endo scopes can acquire high levels of microbial contamination during routine use. A re view of health care–associated infections linked to flexible endoscopes through Jul 1992 found 281 instances of pathogen transmission (ranging from asymptomatic colonization to death) transmitted by gastrointestinal endoscopy and 96 by bron choscopy; a recent review found 130 outbreaks of infections associated with gastro intestinal endoscopes and bronchoscopes, more than any other semicritical medica devices.[1,2]

Endoscopes must be reprocessed between each patient use to ensure they are clean and free from debris and infectious material, decreasing the risk of transmission of pathogens. Reprocessing is a multistep process consisting of cleaning followed b disinfection or sterilization. Cleaning is the physical removal of foreign material (eg, so and organic material), typically using water under pressure, brushes, and detergent: or enzymatic products. High-level disinfection is the elimination of many or all patho genic microorganisms, except large numbers of bacterial spores, typically using liqui chemicals or wet pasteurization. Sterilization eliminates all pathogenic microorgan isms, including bacterial spores, typically using a combination of heat, pressure and time in steam-, gas-, or plasma-based systems. Medical devices are classified as critical, semicritical, or noncritical based on the intended function in a clinical pro cedure according to the Spaulding Classification Scheme, which also determine reprocessing requirements.[3,4] Reusable flexible endoscopes are generally classified as semicritical devices because they contact mucous membranes or nonintact skin conferring a high risk of infection. These should be cleaned and high-level disinfected or cleaned and sterilized after each patient use: if there is an available sterilization pro cess, cleaning and sterilization is preferred.

Device manufacturer instructions for use (IFU) outline the Food and Drug Adminis tration (FDA)-approved methods of reprocessing. Thorough cleaning is the essentia first step in reprocessing to reduce the burden of microbes and soil; failure to adequately perform cleaning and high-level disinfection has been identified in severa investigations of bacterial pathogen transmission associated with these devices.[5–] Cleaning flexible endoscopes is challenging because of their intricate designs and delicate materials. Cleaning and high-level disinfection may be automated or manual Automated endoscope reprocessors are associated with better adherence to recom mended cleaning steps.[9]

In recent years, several accessories or modifications have been introduced to reduce the bioburden on endoscopes or to improve reprocessing, including removable endcaps, cover products, single-use buttons, and other single-use components. Note that endoscope accessories that enter sterile tissue (eg, biopsy forceps) are themselves considered critical devices and should always be sterilized after each patient use. If these endoscope accessories cannot be sterilized after each use, they should be considered single-use items and discarded after use. Lubricating sprays, simethicone, and other accessories that are not approved for use on these devices may contribute to reprocessing failure.[10]

CDC resources relevant to flexible endoscopes include the Guideline for Disinfection and Sterilization in Healthcare Facilities,[3] the Essential Elements of a Reprocessing Program for Flexible Endoscopes – The Recommendations of the HICPAC,[11] and the FDA/CDC/American Society for Microbiology Duodenoscope Surveillance Sampling & Culturing Protocols[12] (discussed in Shanil P. Haugen's article, "Reducing the Risk of Infection from Reprocessed Duodenoscopes – Recent Actions by the U. S. Food and Drug Administration," elsewhere in this issue).

OUTBREAKS AND REPROCESSING LAPSES ARE OPPORTUNITIES TO IDENTIFY DEVICE CONCERNS

Health care facilities are required to report potential outbreaks of infectious diseases to their local or state health department. They may also request assistance in investigating these events, which can include responding to the spread of pathogens in a patient population or evaluating infection risks associated with failure to adhere to reprocessing protocols that remove and inactivate infectious material on reusable medical devices. State and local health departments work with health care facilities to conduct outbreak investigations, coordinate patient notifications and laboratory testing, and recommend control measures. In turn, public health partners may contact CDC for technical assistance to help establish priorities, focus resources, and review findings. CDC can also provide laboratory support in the context of an investigation to confirm species identification, determine antimicrobial susceptibility patterns, identify antibiotic resistance elements, perform molecular typing of clinical samples, and analyze isolates from patient specimens and environmental samples to determine genetic relatedness. The agency can provide onsite technical assistance when requested by the state or local health department, including gathering and interpreting epidemiology, reviewing infection prevention and control practices, and providing laboratory support. CDC also collaborates with other federal agencies, notably the FDA for issues related to medical products and the Center for Medicare and Medicaid Services for issues related to facility regulations and oversight.

CDC has assisted in many outbreak investigations that highlight the transmission risks associated with duodenoscopes and other flexible endoscopes.[5] Some common themes of endoscope-related outbreaks and infection control lapses include complex device design leading to contamination and poor adherence to IFUs or recommended reprocessing practices.[5,8,13] Additionally, problems with reprocessing equipment have been implicated in outbreaks, such as internal contamination of automated endoscope reprocessors and with water of poor quality used for rinsing devices following high-level disinfection.[14]

Findings from endoscope-related outbreaks have driven manufacturer initiatives aimed to reduce the risk of pathogen transmission associated with flexible endoscope use and changes in FDA oversight of these devices, including:

- Refinements in device design

- Enhancements in the design of reprocessing equipment
- Improved environmental standards in health care settings
- Improving reprocessing instructions and protocols taking into consideration real-world performance of reprocessing staff ("human factors")
- Increased recognition of the importance of robust training and adherence to reprocessing protocols

Following the identification in 2013 of the association between duodenoscopes and transmission of multidrug-resistant bacteria,[8] with transmission often related to identified reprocessing deficiencies, much attention has focused on duodenoscopes. Additionally, pathogen transmission events continue to be reported in connection with these devices, including in settings without device damage or failure to adhere to recommended reprocessing instructions, suggesting that residual contamination may remain even after following all manufacturer steps for reprocessing, highlighting a need for additional solutions to reduce risks to patients.[15,16] Other types of gastrointestinal flexible endoscopes may also be susceptible to such issues.

LESSONS LEARNED IN THE LABORATORY

The CDC laboratory has supported numerous endoscope-related outbreak investigations. CDC laboratory support begins with discussion of the relevant epidemiology to inform common exposures among patients, followed by developing testing and sampling strategies in consultation with public health partners. Microbiologists have cultured duodenoscopes, colonoscopes, and endoscopic ultrasound devices for the detection of pathogens and compared recovered pathogens with patient isolates using next-generation sequencing to determine and confirm the causality of transmission from contaminated devices. Laboratory staff have also provided guidance to public health and clinical partners in assessment of endoscope damage and reprocessing practices and collection of related samples.

The FDA, CDC, and the American Society for Microbiology, together with duodenoscope manufacturers and other experts, developed standardized protocols for duodenoscope surveillance sampling and culturing. The protocol is intended for surveillance sampling and quality assurance testing of reprocessed duodenoscopes, and not necessarily for outbreak investigations; however, it can be adapted to maximize the recovery of causative outbreak pathogens at the discretion and capacity of the health care facility.[12] The protocol provides sample collection methods for the instrument channel from biopsy port to distal end using a flush/brush/flush method (FBF) and from the elevator recess by flushing and brushing. Options for culturing endoscope samples are also provided and are limited to detection of high-concern pathogens for surveillance and causative agent of infection. Portions of those protocols can also be used for other devices at the discretion of the health care facility. Based on the culturing methods used (quantitative or presence/absence), the protocol also provides examples of microbial limits, interpretations and response guidance for different levels and presence of high-concern organisms and low/moderate-concern organisms. Selective media and differential media may also be used to detect causative or high-concern agents. Examples of high-concern organisms include gram-negative rods (eg, *Escherichia coli*, *Klebsiella pneumoniae*, other Enterobacteriaceae, and *Pseudomonas aeruginosa*), gram-positive organisms (eg, *Staphylococcus aureus*, β-hemolytic *Streptococcus*, and *Enterococcus* species), and yeasts. In one study, high-concern organisms were identified on 15% of reprocessed duodenoscopes.[17] As of December 2018, FDA had identified upwards of a 6% reprocessing failure rate.[18]

Recovery of an organism by culture methods is highly variable. Flushing alone is not adequate to remove organisms attached to the interior surfaces of duodenoscopes or other flexible endoscopes with ports or channels. Two-thirds of all CDC-processed duodenoscopes, all sampled by FBF, yielded high-concern organisms undetected by prior sampling. In one investigation, high-concern bacteria were detected on a duodenoscope with a total microbial count of 18 colony-forming units (CFU); reprocessing failure is indicated by greater than or equal to one high-concern organism, or 100 CFU or low/moderate-concern organisms. In another instance, the target organism was detected only when total counts exceeded 470 CFU. The FBF method does not guarantee recovery of the target organism but it may reveal another pathogen, which may also suggest that reprocessing failure occurred.[15] Microbial growth should be identified to differentiate high-concern organisms from low/moderate-concern organisms. One or more colonies of a high-concern organism exceeds the microbial limit and indicates a reprocessing failure requiring removal of the endoscope from use.

For duodenoscopes not meant to return to service, destructive processing yields greater recovery of total microbial counts and target organisms, such as in the recovery of New Delhi metallo-β-lactamase-producing carbapenem-resistant E $coli$ from a duodenoscope.[8] In one investigation, three duodenoscopes were sampled using the FBF method, then destructively sampled using bath sonication of the distal tip submerged in a specimen cup containing saline. The total number of recovered organisms from sonication was either equal to or nearly three orders of magnitude greater than the FBF, despite being performed after FBF. Neither method identified the target organism, carbapenem-resistant P $aeruginosa$, at the lowest microbial burden: it was detected only by sonication at a microbial burden of 10^4 CFU; detection by FBF and sonication occurred at the greatest detected burden of 10^6 CFU.

The distal tip of all submitted endoscopes may also be examined for any damage that may retain organic matter and microbes. Using a lens with a $\times 10$ magnification can reveal flaws that would be missed by unaided visual examination, such as chips on the edges of glass lenses (**Fig. 1**). Borescopes may be required to identify kinks or damage within endoscope channels. These flaws can interfere with high-level disinfection and may cause false-negative culture results.

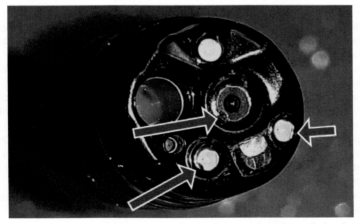

Fig. 1. Distal end of a colonoscope. *Arrows* indicate chips on the edges of glass lenses, which may contribute to reprocessing failure. Using a lens with a $\times 10$ magnification can reveal flaws that would be missed by unaided visual examination.

ACTIONS TO REDUCE ENDOSCOPE-RELATED PATHOGEN TRANSMISSION RISKS

Duodenoscopes are an important source of device-related transmission events, and other reusable gastrointestinal flexible endoscopes may also be susceptible to contamination and subsequent pathogen transmission. Despite recent improvements in device design, reprocessing methods and equipment, and staff training and oversight, pathogen transmission from persistent contamination of flexible gastrointestinal endoscopes continues to occur.[15,16,19] Several factors can contribute to persistent contamination, including intricate device designs that are difficult to clean and disinfect, highly complex reprocessing instructions that are difficult to follow, rapid turnover of endoscopes between procedures leading to reduced time for reprocessing, contamination of the health care environment (including water distribution systems and reprocessing equipment), frequent staff turnover, and inadequate staff training.

Health care facilities can take steps to reduce the risks of transmission events through protocols and training that support adherence to guidelines and manufacturer instructions. In addition, tracking and logging of device use and reprocessing, regular maintenance, and staff training and oversight can support better device maintenance practices, ensure adequate reprocessing of all devices (including loaned devices, which are often not tracked as well as owned devices), and facilitate investigations in the event of pathogen transmission or an infection control lapse. If pathogen transmission might be linked to use of a flexible endoscope, a comprehensive response is warranted to evaluate the device handling and reprocessing to detect lapses in infection control or other issues that contribute to persistent contamination and transmission of infections.

Recently, CDC asked the HICPAC to provide guidance on ways to improve facility-level training and ensure competency for reprocessing of flexible endoscopes. The Essential Elements of a Reprocessing Program for Flexible Endoscopes – Recommendations of the HICPAC, freely available on the Internet, provides minimum expectations for a reprocessing program.[11]

The HICPAC recommendations review essential steps for flexible endoscope reprocessing:

1. *Precleaning* of flexible endoscopes and accessories immediately after finishing a procedure
2. *Leak testing* after each use, and before manual cleaning, which can help identify damage to external surfaces or channels that can lead to persistent contamination or to further damage
3. *Manual cleaning*, including brushing and flushing channels and ports, before performing high-level disinfection or sterilization
4. *Visual inspection* of the endoscope and accessories to ensure these are clean and free of defects: lighted magnification or other methods may be needed for this step
5. *Disinfection or sterilization* with close attention to the manufacturer IFU
6. *Storage* of the endoscope and accessories in a manner that prevents recontamination, protects these items from damage, and promotes drying, either vertically in a cabinet that prevents coiling and touching of the bottom, or horizontally in a unit designed for this purpose
7. *Documentation* of adherence to essential steps each time the endoscope is reprocessed

The HICPAC recommendations also describe key elements for a reprocessing program:

1. *Administrative*, including roles and responsibilities of facility leadership and management and topics to address in policies, including the selection, use, transport, reprocessing, and storage of endoscopes and accessory devices and the management of "loaner" endoscopes
2. *Documentation* of endoscope and patient identifiers, procedure end time, manual cleaning start time, effectiveness of cleaning and disinfection products, preventive maintenance and repair of endoscopes and reprocessing equipment, and investigation of critical or potential critical events
3. *Inventory* of all endoscopes and their reprocessing methods, including each device's unique identifier, manufacturer and model, locations of use, number of procedures, IFU, reprocessing locations and reprocessing equipment used, and current device status
4. *Physical setting* of the reprocessing areas, including a work flow that facilitates separation of clean and dirty; appropriate directional airflow, heating, ventilation, and air conditioning; access to a dedicated handwashing sink, eyewash stations, available IFU; and space to access hardcopy or electronic documentation
5. *Education and training* covering the rationale for the seven essential steps described previously; decontamination, cleaning, and sterilization of certain accessories; training and competency assessment based on each device's IFU and its associated reprocessing equipment and chemicals; and *competency assessment* of trainers, managers, and staff
6. *Risk assessment* or comprehensive gap analysis covering precleaning and transport, reprocessing, staff competencies, sufficient reprocessing personnel for routine and emergency situations, documentation that any automated endoscope reprocessors in use are validated for the endoscopes that they reprocess, and periodic audits of protocols and documentation to monitor compliance
7. Review of every *disinfection/sterilization breach or failure* to determine the risk of transmission of infection to patients and determine the need for notification of patients, in consultation with an infection preventionist and state and local health departments, and to determine the need to report an increase in infections or device contamination to MedWatch, the FDA Safety Information and Adverse Event Reporting program

The HICPAC document also reviews several unresolved issues related to supplemental reprocessing measures, storage interval, storage space, and replacement of endoscopes. Other accompanying materials, all freely available on the CDC Web site, include a policy template, audit tool, competency verification tool, inventory and repair and maintenance log, gap analysis tool, and root cause analysis template, which can be modified for facility use.

Facilities that identify problems with devices or reprocessing instructions should contact the manufacturer and FDA because these findings may have implications for other users and could indicate the need for changes in device design or instructions. Health care facilities should ensure adherence to applicable state and local regulations. Industry guidance for maintaining the safety of the water supply used for reprocessing is found in Association for the Advancement of Medical Instrumentation TIR 34: water quality for the reprocessing of medical devices.[20] Industry guidance and guidelines related to flexible endoscope reprocessing include American National Standards Institute/Association for the Advancement of Medical Instrumentation ST91: comprehensive guide to flexible and semirigid endoscope processing in health care facilities[21] and the 2011 multisociety guideline on reprocessing flexible gastrointestinal endoscopes.[22]

Box 1
Suggested steps before use of a flexible endoscope after possible pathogen transmission or identification of infection control lapse

1. Review device reprocessing instructions, policies, protocols, and practices
   a. Ensure facility has updated manufacturer IFU, including any manufacturer letters that supplement the IFU
   b. Identify other applicable industry or professional society guidelines and applicable state and local regulations
   c. Review facility protocol for reprocessing (cleaning and disinfection, or cleaning and sterilization) to ensure it adheres to manufacturer IFU
      i. If the device is reprocessed using high-level disinfection and there is an available sterilization option, consider a change to sterilization
   d. Device reprocessing should be observed and audited by an individual with working knowledge of reprocessing practices to ensure these adhere to facility protocols
   e. If an automated endoscope reprocessor is used, ensure it is maintained according to manufacturer IFU, including changing enzymatic solution and high-level disinfectant at recommended intervals, checking disinfectant concentration, and logging results
   f. Ensure water for reprocessing adheres to applicable state and local regulations and industry recommendations
   g. Address gaps between policies and practices; report concerns related to IFU to the manufacturer and FDA

2. If device is suspected to have transmitted a pathogen, consider culturing endoscope to determine if contamination is still present
   a. Develop a sampling plan, recognizing that ports, channels, caps, lenses, and moving parts (eg, elevator mechanism, removable caps) are among the most likely areas of damage and microbial colonization
   b. Use flush-brush-flush sampling of ports and channels to maximize opportunities to recover organisms (for duodenoscopes, refer to FDA/CDC/American Society for Microbiology Duodenoscope Surveillance Sampling & Culturing Protocols[12]); if device will not be placed back in use, consider destructive sampling methods for greater recovery of organisms
   c. Await the results of cultures of the devices before placing the devices back into use

3. If contamination persists after reviewing policies and practices, consider sending endoscope to manufacturer for maintenance and to evaluate for damage or defects
   a. Manufacturer evaluation may identify areas of the device, such as kinks or tears to interior channels, that could become colonized and lead to transmission
   b. Ensure manufacturer is aware of possible transmission and concern about device damage and any specific concerns regarding device functionality possibly related to colonization or transmission
   c. Ensure any damage is repaired before placing the device back into use
   d. Consider a review of device handling and storage practices to identify possible sources of damage and opportunities to prevent further damage in the future

4. Consider the role of patient notification and follow-up related to transmission of infection or a lapse in infection control, and the role of reporting information to FDA
   a. Facility personnel and public health authorities should review findings to determine whether there was a deviation from expected practice or persistent contamination that might have placed patients at risk
   b. Strongly consider notifying exposed patients when there is a potential risk of harm, including the possibility of transmission of bloodborne pathogens (human immunodeficiency virus, hepatitis B virus, and hepatitis C virus)[23]
   c. In transmission events involving multidrug-resistant organisms, facility personnel and public health authorities may choose to notify a subset of patients for the purpose of multidrug-resistant organism screening
   d. If a health care provider suspects persistent bacterial contamination of an endoscope following reprocessing, either because of an increase in infections after endoscopic procedures or because of the results of microbiologic culturing of endoscopes, the health care provider should file a voluntary report through MedWatch, the FDA Safety Information and Adverse Event Reporting program

If transmission of a pathogen is suspected to be linked to a flexible endoscope, or an infection control lapse is identified, the health care facility should investigate to identify other potentially affected patients and review device reprocessing IFU, policies, protocols, and practices to ensure adherence to the IFU and other best practices (**Box 1**). Health care facilities may consider culturing the endoscope to determine whether contamination is persistent and, if so, may consider sending the device to the manufacturer to evaluate for damage or defects that could predispose to ongoing contamination. If a reprocessing deficiency is identified, health care facilities should strongly consider notifying the affected patients.[23] Health care facilities should be aware of state requirements for reporting outbreaks to public health authorities and should be familiar with the resources from public health partners for the investigation and control of infections and infection control deficiencies.

THE CONTAINMENT STRATEGY TO IDENTIFY AND CONTAIN NOVEL MULTIDRUG-RESISTANT ORGANISMS

Several transmission events associated with flexible endoscopes were initially detected because of identification of rare, multidrug-resistant organisms. In 2017, CDC outlined an effort to respond rapidly to novel multidrug-resistant organisms; this approach encourages health care facilities and public health authorities to respond to single isolates of an emerging antibiotic-resistant pathogen. That strategy, known as containment, is a systematic response to identify and contain novel multidrug-resistant organisms.[24]

If patients with highly antibiotic-resistant pathogens are identified and endoscopy is determined to be a possible route of transmission, health care personnel and public health authorities should review and enforce adherence to cleaning and disinfection of the endoscope and should review other infection control measures. Repeat assessment should be performed to ensure that infection control gaps are fully addressed. In consultation with public health authorities, health care facility personnel could consider microbiologic culturing of the reprocessed endoscope, depending on the procedure and the duration and type of endoscope. Additionally, a close inspection of the endoscope is warranted. If pathogens are identified from a reprocessed endoscope, the endoscope should be reprocessed and cultured again. Persistently positive endoscopes should be evaluated for damage by the manufacturer. Patients exposed to endoscopes contaminated with highly resistant pathogens should be notified and considered for screening.[12] Culturing of endoscopes to identify contamination with resistant pathogens could also be considered for endoscopes used within 30 days for patients found to be colonized or infected with a highly resistant pathogen for whom exposure to endoscopy is their only health care exposure.

SUMMARY

Gastrointestinal flexible endoscopes are complex devices used to perform essential diagnostic and therapeutic functions in health care settings. These devices are often exposed to high microbial burdens, are reused for many patients, and are difficult to reprocess adequately between patients because of their complex designs, increasing the risk of transmitting pathogens to patients. Research continues to demonstrate the presence of biologic material on reprocessed duodenoscopes and other flexible endoscopes and transmission of pathogens in settings without observed deficiencies in reprocessing, highlighting the continued need to improve the current state of flexible endoscope design and reprocessing.

REFERENCES

1. Spach DH, Silverstein FE, Stamm WE. Transmission of infection by gastrointestinal endoscopy and bronchoscopy. Ann Intern Med 1993;118(2):117–28.
2. Rutala WA, Weber DJ. Reprocessing semicritical items: outbreaks and current issues. Am J Infect Control 2019;47S:A79–89.
3. Rutala WA, Weber DJ, the Healthcare Infection Control Practices Advisory Committee. Guideline for disinfection and sterilization in healthcare facilities, 2008 Update: May 2019. Available at: https://www.cdc.gov/infectioncontrol/guidelines/disinfection/.
4. Spaulding EH. Chemical disinfection of medical and surgical materials. In: Lawrence C, Block SS, editors. Disinfection, sterilization, and preservation. Philadelphia: Lea & Febiger; 1968. p. 517–31.
5. Archibald LK, Jarvis WR. Health care-associated infection outbreak investigations by the Centers for Disease Control and Prevention, 1946-2005. Am J Epidemiol 2011;174(Suppl):S47–64.
6. Agerton T, Valway S, Gore B, et al. Transmission of a highly drug-resistant strain (Strain W1) of *Mycobacterium tuberculosis*: community outbreak and nosocomial transmission via a contaminated bronchoscope. JAMA 1997;278:1073–7.
7. Weldelboe AM, Baumbach J, Blossom DB, et al. Outbreak of cystoscopy related infections with *Pseudomonas aeruginosa*. J Urol 2008;180:588–92.
8. Epstein L, Hunter JC, Arwady MA. New Delhi metallo-β-lactamase-producing carbapenem-resistant *Escherichia coli* associated with exposure to duodenoscopes. JAMA 2014;312(14):1447–55.
9. Ofstead CL, Wetzler HP, Snyder AK, et al. Endoscope reprocessing methods: a prospective study on the impact of human factors and automation. Gastroenterol Nurs 2010;33(4):304–11.
10. Ofstead CL, Hopkins KM, Eiland JE, et al. Widespread clinical use of simethicone, insoluble lubricants, and tissue glue during endoscopy: a call to action for infection preventionists. Am J Infect Control 2019;47(6):666–70.
11. Healthcare Infection Control Practices Advisory Committee (HICPAC). Essential elements of a reprocessing program for flexible endoscopes: the recommendations of the Healthcare Infection Control Practices Advisory Committee (HICPAC). 2016 Available at: https://www.cdc.gov/hicpac/pdf/flexible-endoscope-reprocessing.pdf. Accessed July 22, 2020.
12. U.S. Food and Drug Administration (FDA). Duodenoscope surveillance sampling & culturing: reducing the risk of infection. 2018. Available at: https://www.fda.gov/media/111081/download. Accessed July 22, 2020.
13. CDC. Bronchoscopy-related infections and pseudo-infections—New York, 1996 and 1998. MMWR Morb Mortal Wkly Rep 1999;48(26):557–60.
14. Maloney S, Welbel S, Daves B, et al. *Mycobacterium abscessus* pseudoinfection traced to an automated endoscope washer: utility of epidemiologic and laboratory investigation. J Infect Dis 1994;169(5):1166–9.
15. Shenoy ES, Pierce VM, Walters MS. Transmission of mobile colistin resistance (mcr-1) by duodenoscope. Clin Infect Dis 2019;68(8):1327–34.
16. Wendorf KA, Kay M, Baliga C, et al. Endoscopic retrograde cholangiopancreatography-associated AmpC *Escherichia coli* outbreak. Infect Control Hosp Epidemiol 2015;35(6):634–42.
17. Rauwers AW, Voor In 't Holt AF, Buijs JG. High prevalence rate of digestive tract bacteria in duodenoscopes: a nationwide study. Gut 2018;67(9):1637–45.

18. FDA. The FDA provides interim results of duodenoscope reprocessing studies conducted in real-world settings: FDA Safety Communication. 2018. Available at: https://www.fda.gov/medical-devices/safety-communications/fda-provides-interim-results-duodenoscope-reprocessing-studies-conducted-real-world-settings-fda. Accessed July 22, 2020.
19. FDA. Infections associated with reprocessed duodenoscopes. 2019. Available at: https://www.fda.gov/medical-devices/reprocessing-reusable-medical-devices/infections-associated-reprocessed-duodenoscopes. Accessed July 22, 2020.
20. Association for the Advancement of Medical Instrumentation (AAMI). Water quality for the reprocessing of medical devices. AAMI TIR 34:2014. Arlington (VA): AAMI; 2014. Available at: https://my.aami.org/store/detail.aspx?id=TIR34-PDF. Accessed July 22, 2020.
21. AAMI. ANSI/AAMI ST91: Comprehensive guide to flexible and semi-rigid endoscope processing in health care facilities. 2015. Available at: https://www.aami.org/productspublications/ProductDetail.aspx?ItemNumber=2477. Accessed July 22, 2020.
22. American Society for Gastrointestinal Endoscopy (ASGE), Petersen BT, Chennat J, et al. Multisociety guideline on reprocessing flexible gastrointestinal endoscopes: 2011. Gastrointest Endosc 2011;73(6):1075–84. Available at: https://www.giejournal.org/article/S0016-5107(11)01419-2/abstract. Accessed July 22, 2020.
23. Patel PR, Srinivasan A, Perz JP. Developing a broader approach to management of infection control breaches in health care settings. Am J Infect Control 2008; 36(10):685–90.
24. CDC. Interim guidance for a public health response to contain novel or targeted multidrug-resistant organisms (MDROs). 2019. Available at: https://www.cdc.gov/hai/pdfs/containment/Health-Response-Contain-MDRO-H.pdf. Accessed July 22, 2020.

Outbreak Investigations

A Brief Primer for Gastroenterologists

nnabelle de St. Maurice, MD, MPH[a,b], Zachary A. Rubin, MD[c],*

KEYWORDS

- Outbreak investigations • Outbreak communications • Endoscope-related outbreaks

KEY POINTS

- Endoscope-related outbreak investigations are best undertaken by multidisciplinary teams that include gastroenterologists.
- Endoscope-related outbreaks are difficult to identify, so gastroenterologists should work with local infection prevention and laboratory staff to design surveillance systems to pro-actively identify endoscope-related outbreaks early.
- Managing outbreak-related communication is the most critical part of the investigation for the reputation of an institution and gastroenterologists can help greatly improve this communication.

INTRODUCTION

Over the last decade there have been several high-profile outbreak investigations that ultimately identified the transmission of multidrug-resistant nosocomial bacterial in-fections related to endoscopes. Hospital and public health epidemiologists have therefore been focused on looking for additional endoscope-related outbreaks and continue to uncover them, despite the Food and Drug Administration (FDA)-recom-mended additional steps to prevent potential transmissions.[1] There is a high likelihood that these outbreaks will continue until definitive changes to duodenoscope design are made in the future. It is therefore important that gastroenterologists (GIs) become familiar not only with the problems and potential preventative actions (discussed else-where in this issue), but that they should also be generally familiar with how to work with outbreak investigators to successfully navigate their institution through an inves-tigation. It is true that outbreak investigations are typically the purview of the hospital epidemiology physicians and staff in health care infection prevention, but GIs are crit-ical to the success of any investigation of endoscope-related infections. Not only do

[a] UCLA Division of Infectious Diseases, Department of Pediatrics, 22-442 MDCC, 10833 Le Conte Avenue, Los Angeles, CA 90095-1752, USA; [b] Department of Pediatrics, David Geffen School of Medicine at UCLA, 924 Westwood Boulevard, Suite 900, Los Angeles, CA 90095, USA; [c] Acute Communicable Disease Control, Los Angeles County Department of Public Health, 313 North Figueroa Street, Room 212, Los Angeles, CA 90012, USA
* Corresponding author.
E-mail address: zrubin@ph.lacounty.gov

Gastrointest Endoscopy Clin N Am 30 (2020) 735–743
https://doi.org/10.1016/j.giec.2020.06.006   giendo.theclinics.com

GIs and their staff understand the local processes within the endoscopy suite making them important sources of information, they also add great value as communicators with their patients, their health care colleagues, and the general public. In our opinion GIs should be intimately involved in the notification of patients and staff and educating the public and other health care providers about potential outbreaks and the routine risks related to endoscopy procedures.

Although this article is not intended to be a definitive discussion of outbreak investigations, it was written as a practical guide to some of the important aspects of outbreak investigations for GI physicians. The specific areas in which GIs can take a central role are emphasized: the initial identification of an outbreak, patient notification, and internal and external communications plans.

WHAT IS AN OUTBREAK INVESTIGATION?

An outbreak is defined as a "significant" increase of some event over the background rate of that event.[2] The main objective of outbreak investigations is to confirm the presence of a significant increase in rate over the baseline and then to identify risk factors and commonalities among cases to prevent further transmission.[2,3] Clinicians should suspect an outbreak if health care workers and patients have similar infections particularly with multidrug resistant organisms (MDROs), and if a cluster of similar infections is associated with a particular geographic unit or invasive device.[2] The steps of an outbreak investigation are highlighted in **Table 1**. Perhaps the most challenging aspect of an outbreak investigation is creating a case definition. The purpose of a case definition is to be able to systematically count outbreak cases in an objective manner. If the case definition is too narrow, you may not capture all of the cases and draw incorrect conclusions. If the definition is too broad, you may not be able to pinpoint a common exposure. As you collect more data, you will need to revise the case definition to improve accuracy. Once a case definition has been agreed on, the next step is creating a line-list and finding cases. A line-list should be organized so that similarities between cases are easily identified. As more data are collected, hypotheses should be tested usually using cohort or case-control studies and appropriate control measures should be implemented to control the spread of disease.

Outbreak investigations require a multidisciplinary team including clinicians, microbiology, nursing, and infection prevention.[2] Depending on the extent of the outbreak, it may be necessary to create a hospital emergency incident command center.[2] This center is used to create a structure for emergency response to assign roles for hospital leadership, risk management, physicians, nurses, ancillary staff, and media relations/communications. Even if your organization decides not to implement an incident command center, it is still important to have a multidisciplinary team that can address regulatory, media, technical, legal, and clinical concerns in a timely manner.

Clear communication with the public health department and other agencies is important because they can help with the investigation and prevent further infections at other sites. Each state has different reporting requirements for hospital-acquired infections and may handle outbreaks slightly differently. However, all states require timely reporting of potential outbreaks to public health authorities. Failure to report outbreak investigations can result in a reprimand or even legal action by authorities and can lead to additional infections if the underlying cause of the outbreak is not quickly remediated. The FDA created an Internet-based reporting system for all device-related concerns called MedSun.[4] Users can search and report medical device-related concerns to the FDA using this Web site (https://www.accessdata.fda.gov/scripts/cdrh/cfdocs/Medsun/searchreport.cfm).   Failure

Table 1
Steps in an outbreak investigation

	Notes
1. Confirm the existence of an outbreak	Compare the current number of cases with the baseline Consider artifactual reasons for an increase in cases caused by changes in surveillance practices, diagnostic methods, or changes in practice
2. Confirm the diagnosis	Review laboratory and clinical records
3. Identify and count cases	Create a case definition Find cases by reviewing laboratory records and diagnoses, contacting clinicians and laboratory directors Create a line-list
4. Organize the data by person, place, and time	Characterize affected individuals by age, comorbidities, recent health care exposures/procedures Plot an epidemic curve, number of cases over time, to better visualize the spread and duration of the outbreak Create maps or figures demonstrating location of the outbreak
5. Identify who is at risk	Review risk factors of cases and line-list
6. Create a hypothesis	Develop a hypothesis of disease transmission based on identification of risk factors
7. Test the hypothesis and compare with existing data	Use statistical methods to assess whether the hypothesis is plausible Compare the hypothesis with established facts and existing data
8. Plan a more systematic study	Consider conducting case-control or cohort studies to answer additional questions and revise the case definition
9. Implement control measures	Using the data collected address risk factors to prevent further disease
10. Prepare a written report	Communicate findings to leadership and public health authorities Written communications can serve as a document for medical or legal purposes Can be used to educate others on risk factors

Adapted from: Gregg, MB. Conducting a Field Investigation. In: Gregg, MB. Field Epidemiology 3rd edition. New York: Oxford University Press; 2008. p. 83-96; Jarvis, WR. Investigation of Outbreaks. In: Mayhall, CG. Hospital Epidemiology and Infection Control 4th edition. Philadelphia: Lippincott Williams and Wilkins; 2012. P126-141; Goodman RA, Buehler JW, Koplan JP. The epidemiologic field investigation: science and judgement in public health practice. Am J Epidemiology 1990; 132:9-16; with permission.

to report infections to these FDA systems can also result in potential legal action, so it is important to report.

IDENTIFICATION OF AN OUTBREAK

Although outbreak investigations can progress quickly based on well-established steps as described previously, the initial identification of an outbreak is challenging and depends on practice setting and resources available. Surveillance for possible outbreaks should be ongoing. Surveillance methodologies are separated into active and passive surveillance. The most comprehensive scheme, but also the most labor-intensive type of surveillance, is using a standardized, electronic surveillance system similar to the Centers for Disease Control and Prevention's National Healthcare Safety Network (NHSN) system for surgical site infections.[5] Although there are several clear benefits to this type of active surveillance system, the current lack of an NHSN module to support the effort and the considerable effort to set up and maintain the system limit its use at this time.

Although using NHSN-like active surveillance for endoscope-related infections should be considered the gold standard, other active surveillance schemes may be less sensitive, but may still provide important data without as much cost. Identifying bloodstream infections in patients within 30 days of their duodenoscopy has been shown to be somewhat effective.[6,7] This system trades lower sensitivity for greater efficiency and may miss post-procedure infections that are nonbacteremic and limited to intra-abdominal involvement, such as abscesses and cholangitis. Another downside of this strategy is that without clearly defined background rates of bacteremia after endoscopy, it is difficult to identify a trigger for an investigation. Recent studies demonstrate that the baseline rate of positivity may depend on the timing of the blood culture draw after the procedure. For example, the three studies identified[5-7] demonstrated a range of post-procedure bacteremia rates between 1% and 2.2% when blood cultures were drawn only after clinical signs or symptoms and 28% when all patients were cultured 15 minutes after the procedure.

Another type of active surveillance that is possible without building new surveillance infrastructure is to use the existing surveillance for MDROs performed currently by most hospitals. Using these existing systems, investigators would check all MDROs retrospectively for endoscopy procedures within 30 days. This strategy is certainly easier in terms of resources, but would miss clusters of infections because of susceptible organisms or organisms currently not on the MDRO list recommended by Centers for Disease Control and Prevention. It is also not realistic for freestanding endoscopy centers that do not have easy access to microbiology laboratory results.

Surveilling for infections in the outpatient location is more challenging given the lack of electronic connectivity to hospitals that may admit patients after complications. In this setting, postdischarge surveillance with follow-up telephone calls to patients is a possible option. This approach has been used for surgical site infection surveillance, but can result in spurious results if patients provide inaccurate or misleading answers. It is also labor intensive to make these calls, particularly if relying on clinical staff. One option is to use nonclinical staff to make the initial screening call that can then be followed up by clinical staff if a patient answers affirmatively to any questions suggesting a possible complication. Having a standardized script of questions for patients is important if nonclinical staff are making the follow-up calls.

Despite the higher sensitivity of active surveillance, most facilities currently rely on what is considered passive surveillance. Passive surveillance requires the notification of investigators when a potential infection is identified by a clinician or other source. These more anecdotal systems are typically not as reliable as active surveillance systems in identification of outbreaks, but can supplement active systems that may be looking for only a narrow range of infections. The post–endoscopic retrograde cholangiopancreatography outbreak at University of California Los Angeles was identified in this manner when an astute clinician alerted epidemiologists to an unusual case. This observation in turn led to additional investigation and ultimate identification of an outbreak before when it might have been identified through active MDRO

urveillance.[8] However, this approach of relying only on passive surveillance can result
 delayed recognition of outbreaks. This was true in two large outbreaks, which were
entified serendipitously by outside investigators studying MDROs after long de-
ys.[9,10] Even this passive type of surveillance requires outreach to ensure that they
e aware of the requirement and the logistics of reporting.

Whatever surveillance is chosen by a facility, GI physicians should be aware of the
rengths and weaknesses of the system and consider using a combination of
ifferent systems. Short of a gold standard NHSN type of system, the best system
kely includes a combination of techniques: surveillance for bacteremia within the
0 days after endoscopy, MDRO surveillance, and passive notification by clinical staff.

HAT GASTROENTEROLOGISTS SHOULD KNOW ABOUT MOLECULAR
AGNOSTICS

nce a potential cluster of bacterial infections is identified, the next step is typically to
onfirm a point-source outbreak, often using molecular microbiologic testing.
lthough a comprehensive discussion of molecular testing of bacteria is beyond the
cope of this article, it is important for GIs to have a general understanding of the abil-
y of microbiologic techniques to detect relatedness of organisms. Historically, before
cilities had access to many molecular methods of differentiation, investigators often
sed the bacterial antimicrobial resistance pattern to try to estimate relatedness.
lthough analyzing the resistance pattern of organisms is done quickly and easily, it
 not always reliable, especially in the setting of plasmid-mediated resistance that
an shift quickly, making molecular diagnostics more effective in proving relatedness.
ulse field gel electrophoresis (PFGE), which has been relied on as the standard by
pidemiology and public health laboratories for decades, analyzes the genomic
NA of organisms and compares the patterns made when restriction enzymes cut
NA into fragments that are run on an agar gel, forming band patterns. As whole
enome sequencing (WGS) has become more widely available, it has been noted
at PFGE is often unable to differentiate between highly clonal organisms, such as
cinetobacter and *Klebsiella*, making WGS a better choice.[11] Although PFGE and
VGS are time and labor intensive, WGS is less subjective than PFGE. Other tech-
iques, such as multiple locus sequence typing and repetitive-element polymerase
hain reaction, can be used,[12] but all have their own strengths and weaknesses.
ecause the cost of WGS has decreased and computing power to run analysis is
ore accessible, the technology is increasingly being implemented in clinical and
ublic health laboratories. WGS has the benefit of being able to identify not only chro-
osomal DNA, but also plasmids and phages. The main limitations of this technique
re cost, availability, and the complexity of the analysis.

Although it is unrealistic for GI investigators to understand the many nuances of mo-
cular epidemiology, it is important for them to ask specific questions about whether
e molecular epidemiology performed is able to correctly characterize a cluster of
acteria as a true outbreak. If your local health department or clinical laboratory
nly has access to PFGE, consider sending the isolates to a laboratory able to perform
VGS for better resolution. Because most laboratories discard bacterial isolates within
 short period, consider asking your clinical laboratory to hold onto resistant bacteria
or a longer time period to make molecular testing feasible.

ATIENT NOTIFICATION

nce an outbreak has been identified and reported to public health authorities, inves-
gators quickly reach the most fraught aspect of an investigation: deciding when and

whether to notify patients and other health care providers of an outbreak. In our expe rience over the last decade of practice as hospital epidemiologists, the approach t notification of patients has changed significantly. Previously, it was not unusual fo health care facilities, in consultation with public health authorities, to determin whether public notification was necessary on an outbreak-by-outbreak basis. Man of these decisions whether to notify were underpinned by the fear of malpractice suit from health care facilities and a paternalistic view that notification itself might result i greater perceived harm to patients than the disease itself.

Over the last decade, however, long-established norms regarding patient and pub lic notification have been changing. Not only are institutions more accustomed to pub lic reporting of hospital-acquired infection rates as mandated by most states, th general public and the press is now more aware of patient safety and outbreak than ever before. Health care facilities are now largely expected by the public an by public health to report outbreaks quickly to affected patients. The perceived failur or delay to report can result in adverse publicity that can compound or overshadov the original outbreak and can erode confidence in an institution.[13]

The public interest in increasing health care transparency is demonstrated in growing scientific literature of patient and physician attitudes toward disclosure.[14,1] In the United States, the need to notify patients still varies depending on public healt jurisdictions, but some countries, such as Canada, have taken steps to further stan dardize the process. There is growing interest in the United States to similarly stan dardize public health reporting guidelines.[16]

The Canadian guidance is consistent with more modern practice statements from individual facilities, requiring patient and public health notification for patient safet events that either harmed or could have seriously harmed patients. When a medica event or outbreak does not actually reach patients directly, such as a "near miss" erro or pseudo-outbreak, there is no strict requirement to notify patients unless there i ongoing risk.

From a practical standpoint, it is often helpful to notify patients early in the investi gation. This is necessary because rumors and misinformation typically start as inves tigators reach out to potentially exposed patients early in the outbreak investigation process. Even when an outbreak is not yet confirmed, patients should be given a basi understanding of the investigation and the potential risks identified. Public notificatior within the facility may be necessary if the source of an outbreak has not been identified so that patients who may be undergoing a procedure under investigation can make fully informed decisions about whether to proceed with the potentially problematic treatment or exposure.

Once the decision has been made to notify patients and the public, our experienc suggests that it is important to have a written notification plan before contacting pa tients. The notification plan should include the specific patient population to be noti fied, timeframe and a script. If possible, patients should be verbally notified by patient's own health care provider. It may be helpful to include one of the investigators more versed in the logistics of the investigation who can then answer more technica questions. Plans for follow-up testing or visits should be made for the patient at th time of contact. Any charges related to the testing should be covered by the healt care facility if possible. In our experience, it is important to send written, dated letters to patients explaining the exposure, even if verbal notification is given. Attachin frequently asked questions written in accessible language with the notification lette is helpful in explaining the situation further to patients. If the notification plan i executed well, it can help patients believe that they are being cared for, even if th health care facility is at fault. Local public health departments are often willing to assis with notifications, but our strong recommendation is that facilities should contact their own patients.

The most important aspect to communicating effectively in the setting of outbreak, in our experience, is to be truthful, contrite, and reassure patients that investigators and clinicians are doing their utmost to address the individual patient's concerns. Furthermore, it is important to highlight that the institution is working with local public health officials to ensure the safety of all patients undergoing treatment in the future. Timely patient notification is important and any delays of notification, even to finalize the medical follow-up, should be avoided because they can undermine patient trust significantly. It is important to keep protected patient information from being divulged unnecessarily, so any information within the verbal or written notification should be careful not to contain any patient identifiers.

INTERNAL AND EXTERNAL COMMUNICATIONS

Paralleling the notification process for patients is the need for facilities to have an internal and external communications plan. Internal communications are designed as inward-facing statements that help health care workers in the facility understand the basics of an investigation without compromising patient privacy. External communications are prepared for the general public and the news media should an investigation become widely known. External communications may also include patients currently in the hospital or under care of the facility that may be affected by an ongoing investigation. All types of communication should be developed with cooperation among GIs, investigators, and media relations or communications staff, if available.

Like patient notification, having an internal communication plan ready at the time of patient notification is helpful. This communication should outline the general facts of the outbreak investigation, but should be careful to avoid any protected patient information and conjecture or theories. Ideally, these statements should also include frequently asked questions that can be used by staff who may be uninvolved in the investigation, but may be queried by patients nonetheless. In our experience, misinformation and rumors spread quickly among staff during outbreak investigations, so timely and accurate communication is critical.

It is helpful to prepare statements that can educate and reassure patients uninvolved with the outbreak or discuss potential options for those patients who may be at risk. Additionally, many public health departments now require written notification of an outbreak investigation be posted in a public place within the facility. Direct notification of patients within the institution who may read the written notification is helpful in ensuring that patients understand the risks of the potential exposure and have the opportunity to ask specific questions about how their care may be impacted. In one recent outbreak at our institution, we posted written material at the nursing unit entry explaining the investigation and the potential risks to patients. The letter had been written by physicians at our institution in collaboration with local health departments. The day the notice was posted, physicians also went to all patients and explained the investigation and provided them a copy of written notification. For the entire duration of the posted written notification, every new admission to the unit was provided the same in-person and written notification. Once the outbreak investigation identified the cause of the problem and remediated the issue, the notification was removed with approval of the local health department. We believe that the additional communication resulted in greater understanding of the actual risks to patients and led to better patient satisfaction compared with a posted notification alone.

With any public notification of an outbreak investigation, there is a significant risk of alerting the news media to a potential story. Once a media outlet starts to work on a story about your investigation, the level of anxiety rises not only for administrators and investigators, but also for uninvolved staff and patients. Having a timely and accurate "holding statement" that is sent in response to inquiries can help insulate investigators from having to spend lots of time interacting with the media. It is also extremely important to send out timely information to patients of your facility who may be concerned about media reports. In our experience, a flood of calls from the worried well can overwhelm an organization and adversely impact patient care. Submitting information proactively to patients via electronic notification systems and mail may help, but it is critical to think proactively. In one very public outbreak at our institution, the department handling telephone calls quickly became overwhelmed after the media reported the outbreak. In response to the large volume of calls, the institution set-up a call center and trained nurses to triage calls, ensuring that truly affected patients could get through to important resources, while uninvolved patients were reassured. After this experience, we develop a detailed communication plan with every outbreak investigation, including the potential to open a staffed hotline number if necessary.

In an endoscope-related outbreak, GIs are likely to be the most knowledgeable and best prepared to help with the development of the communication planning and patient notification. GIs should be a central part of the investigation and should be empowered to participate and ensure that the transmission of information is accurate and timely and reflects the best scientific and logistical information available. GIs can best identify potential treatment and local resources that can help patients address their concerns and seek out helpful medical attention if necessary.

SUMMARY

Although outbreak investigations are stressful for an individual institution, publicizing the outbreak can shed light on a problem and lead to action. In the case of duodenoscope-related outbreaks, we believe the media scrutiny received by well-respected institutions pushed federal agencies to react more forcefully to identified problems from the outbreaks. This greater attention is leading gradually to developing greater safeguards for patients. In this way, although outbreaks can have immediate negative impacts on individual institutions, the public knowledge of these institutions can save lives globally. Institutions, therefore, should aggressively investigate outbreaks and highlight this robust approach to transparency to patients and media. As public health standardizes its approach to publicizing these outbreaks, public notifications will likely become more common. Having a clear institutional goal to address potential outbreaks aggressively is important to reassuring patients and providers that the institution is serious about patient safety. Preemptively developing a plan to notify patients and communicate with staff with the input of a broad team of clinicians ensures that the investigation proceeds smoothly and rapidly.

DISCLOSURE

The authors have nothing to disclose.

REFERENCES

1. Food and Drug Administration. Supplemental measures to enhance duodenoscope reprocessing: FDA safety communication. 2015. Available at: https://

www.fdanews.com/ext/resources/files/08-15/081015-duodenoscopes-fda.pdf? 1520541508. Accessed September 13, 2019.

2. Jarvis W. Investigation of outbreaks. In: Mayhall CG. Hospital epidemiology and infection control. Philadelphia: Lippincott Williams and Wilkins; 2012. p. 126–41.

3. Jarvis WR. Nosocomial outbreaks: the Centers for Disease Control's Hospital Infections Program experience, 1980-1990. Epidemiology Branch, Hospital Infections Program. Am J Med 1991;91(3B):101S–6S.

4. Food and Drug Administration. MedSun: Medical Product Safety Network. 2018. Available at: https://www.fda.gov/medical-devices/medical-device-safety/medsun-medical-product-safety-network. Accessed September 13, 2019.

5. Du M, Suo J, Liu B, et al. Post-ERCP infection and its epidemiological and clinical characteristics in a large Chinese tertiary hospital: a 4-year surveillance study. Antimicrob Resist Infect Control 2017;6:131.

6. Thosani N, Zubarik RS, Kochar R, et al. Prospective evaluation of bacteremia rates and infectious complications among patients undergoing single-operator choledochoscopy during ERCP. Endoscopy 2016;48(5):424–31.

7. Anderson DJ, Shimpi RA, McDonald JR, et al. Infectious complications following endoscopic retrograde cholangiopancreatography: an automated surveillance system for detecting postprocedure bacteremia. Am J Infect Control 2008; 36(8):592–4.

8. Humphries RM, Yang S, Kim S, et al. Duodenoscope-related outbreak of a carbapenem-resistant *Klebsiella pneumoniae* identified using advanced molecular diagnostics. Clin Infect Dis 2017;65(7):1159–66.

9. Epstein L, Hunter JC, Arwady MA, et al. New Delhi metallo-beta-lactamase-producing carbapenem-resistant *Escherichia coli* associated with exposure to duodenoscopes. JAMA 2014;312(14):1447–55.

10. Wendorf KA, Kay M, Baliga C, et al. Endoscopic retrograde cholangiopancreatography-associated AmpC *Escherichia coli* outbreak. Infect Control Hosp Epidemiol 2015;36(6):634–42.

11. Salipante SJ, SenGupta DJ, Cummings LA, et al. Application of whole-genome sequencing for bacterial strain typing in molecular epidemiology. J Clin Microbiol 2015;53(4):1072–9.

12. Sabat AJ, Budimir A, Nashev D, et al. Overview of molecular typing methods for outbreak detection and epidemiological surveillance. Euro Surveill 2013;18(4): 20380.

13. Aleccia J. Undisclosed superbug sickened dozens at Virginia Mason. The Seattle Times 2015.

14. Gallagher TH, Waterman AD, Ebers AG, et al. Patients' and physicians' attitudes regarding the disclosure of medical errors. JAMA 2003;289(8):1001–7.

15. Wu AW, Boyle DJ, Wallace G, et al. Disclosure of adverse events in the United States and Canada: an update, and a proposed framework for improvement. J Public Health Res 2013;2(3):e32.

16. Canadian Patient Safety Institute. 2011. Available at: https://www.patientsafetyinstitute.ca/en/toolsResources/disclosure/Documents/CPSI%20Canadian%20Disclosure%20Guidelines.pdf. Accessed September 9, 2019.

The Endoscopy Patient as a Vector and Victim

Brian P.H. Chan, MD, FRCPC, Tyler M. Berzin, MD*

KEYWORDS

- Endoscopy • Infection • Adverse Events • Prophylaxis

KEY POINTS

- Patient and procedural factors can increase the risk of infectious adverse events during endoscopy.
- Prophylactic antibiotic use must be judicious and individualized in the era of antibiotic resistance.
- New and emerging procedures require high-quality studies to elucidate appropriate risk profiles.

INTRODUCTION

It is estimated that more than 14 million colonoscopies[1] and 20 million gastrointestinal (GI) endoscopic procedures[2] are performed annually in the United States. Despite the large volume of procedures, infectious adverse events during routine endoscopy remain rare. Routine upper endoscopy has a reported rate of transient bacteremia of 3% to 8%,[3–5] and in flexible sigmoidoscopy, the rate is less than 1%.[6] In colonoscopy, with or without polypectomy, transient bacteremia may occur in approximately 4% of cases, with a reported range of 0% to 25%.[7–9] Transient bacteremia can occur with any trauma to a mucosal surface, which is populated with endogenous microflora, and is rarely of clinical significance. Indeed, transient bacteremia can be identified in routine activities from tooth brushing or flossing (20%–68%) to chewing food (7%–51%).[10–12] Although there have been case reports of clinically relevant infection following colonoscopy in noncirrhotic patients, this is considered an extremely rare event, and there is no proven benefit for antibiotic prophylaxis.[13]

Endoscopy-related infections can be categorized as endogenous or exogenous.[6] Endogenous infections are more common during endoscopy and result from the patient's own microbial flora. Exogenous infections involve a pathogen entering the body from the surrounding environment. In endoscopy, this can occur from a contaminated endoscope or from the tools used during endoscopy. This article explores both the

Division of Gastroenterology, Center for Advanced Endoscopy, Beth Israel Deaconess Medical Center, Harvard Medical School, 330 Brookline Avenue, Boston, MA 02215, USA
* Corresponding author.
E-mail address: tberzin@bidmc.harvard.edu

Gastrointest Endoscopy Clin N Am 30 (2020) 745–762
https://doi.org/10.1016/j.giec.2020.06.007
1052-5157/20/© 2020 Elsevier Inc. All rights reserved.

giendo.theclinics.com

endogenous and the exogenous factors that increase the risk of infection during GI endoscopy.

HIGH-RISK PATIENTS

In a subgroup of the population undergoing endoscopy, patient-related risk factors increase the risk of adverse infectious events. In patients with these medical conditions, endoscopy can lead to bacterial translocation into the bloodstream or the introduction of bacteria into previously sterile spaces. Identification of this population and appropriate antibiotic prophylaxis can reduce the risk of endoscopy-related infection. In this section, the patient factors that increase risk of endoscopy-related infections are explored.

High-Risk Cardiac Conditions

In 2007, the American Heart Association (AHA) guideline on prevention of infective endocarditis (IE) recommended against the administration of prophylactic antibiotics solely to prevent IE for most patients undergoing GI endoscopy.[10] The only exception was for patients with specific cardiac conditions at highest risk of an adverse outcome from IE (**Box 1**), who also had a concomitant GI tract infection, in which case an agent active against enterococci was suggested. Although GI tract infections are often polymicrobial, enterococci are most likely to cause IE.

It is worth noting that the previous AHA guideline, published in 1997, recommended broader use of prophylactic antibiotics for GI endoscopy.[14] The newer 2007 AHA recommendations relied on several lines of reasoning: (1) GI endoscopy causes transient bacteremia, but there is no evidence to establish a link between GI endoscopy and IE; (2) cases of IE following GI endoscopy are largely anecdotal; (3) there are no data that demonstrate antibiotic prophylaxis during GI endoscopy prevents IE. Therefore, antibiotic prophylaxis is only suggested in patients with high-risk cardiac conditions (see **Box 1**) with concomitant GI tract infections.

Incomplete Biliary Drainage

Although cholangitis is a primary indication for endoscopic retrograde cholangiopancreatography (ERCP), and successful endoscopic drainage is a cornerstone of cholangitis treatment, cholangitis and sepsis can also occur as a complication of ERCP, in 1% to 3% of cases.[15–18] This risk is increased in patients in whom there is incomplete biliary drainage, such as cases of primary sclerosing cholangitis or patients with

---

Box 1
High-risk cardiac conditions for infective endocarditis

Prosthetic (mechanical or bioprosthetic) cardiac valve

Previous infective endocarditis

Cardiac transplant patients who develop cardiac valvulopathy

Congenital heart disease (CHD)
   Unrepaired CHD, including palliative shunts and conduits
   Completely repaired CHD with prosthetic material or device, whether placed by surgery or catheter intervention during the first 6 months after the procedure
   Repaired CHD with residual defects at the site or adjacent to the site of a prosthetic patch or prosthetic device

lar cholangiocarcinoma.[19,20] In these situations, the introduction of nonsterile bile or ontrast material into an obstructed system can result in biliary sepsis. Current interational guidelines do not recommend the use of prophylactic antibiotics for ERCP in ie absence of cholangitis, unless incomplete biliary drainage is anticipated or recognized during the procedure.[13,21,22]

Three metaanalyses have been performed to determine the role of prophylactic anoiotics in patients undergoing elective ERCP (**Table 1**).[23–25] The study reported by ai and colleagues[24] included 2 trials published after the analysis reported by Harris nd colleagues,[23] whereas the most recent Cochrane review[25] had an overlap of 6 tudies. In the Harris and Bai metaanalyses, the trials did not include high-risk patients ith predicted incomplete drainage. In contrast to the previous metaanalyses, the ochrane analysis found the use of prophylactic antibiotics was significantly favored) prevent cholangitis, septicemia, bacteremia, and pancreatitis. However, there was) benefit for prophylactic antibiotics in the subgroup of patients with complete clearnce and adequate drainage of the bile duct.

A retrospective analysis of 11,484 ERCPs over an 11-year period was conducted to ssess the role of antibiotic prophylaxis.[26] Over the course of 11 years, the use of antiiotic prophylaxis was sequentially reduced, starting with 95% of patients receiving ntibiotics, and progressing to antibiotic administration only in patients in whom icomplete biliary drainage was suspected. During this time, antibiotic use was educed from greater than 90% of procedures (3154 patients), to 46% (1882 patients), nd finally to 26% (1050 patients). In each period, the overall number of patients was imilar. There was a low overall infection rate, which decreased from 0.48% to 0.25% ver time. Patients undergoing ERCP for biliary conditions after liver transplantation rere determined to be high risk for infection in multivariate analysis. In summary, prohylactic antibiotics for patients undergoing ERCP should be limited to those in whom icomplete biliary drainage is expected or noted during the procedure. Although any atient may have transient bacteremia resulting from ERCP, this rarely leads to sepsis r cholangitis.

uodenoscope Transmitted Infections

here has been increasing concern regarding duodenoscope-related transmission of iultidrug-resistant organisms. The duodenoscope is among the most complex med:al instruments to undergo disinfection between patients, with the elevator channel eing a unique feature that increases the risk of biofilm formation and incomplete isinfection.[27] A recent study from the Netherlands using a threshold of $\geq$20 olony-forming units of microorganisms showed that 15% of patient-ready duodenocopes were contaminated.[28] In 2018, there were several deaths reported in the nited States related to duodenoscope-transmitted infection,[29] bringing renewed

Table 1
Summary of metaanalyses on antibiotic prophylaxis to prevent post-endoscopic retrograde cholangiopancreatography cholangitis in elective endoscopic retrograde cholangiopancreatography

Metaanalysis, Year	Randomized Clinical Trials Included	Total Patients	Prophylaxis Benefit
Harris et al,[23] 1999	5	1029	No
Bai et al,[24] 2009	7	1389	No
Brand et al,[25] 2010	9	1573	Yes

focus on the adequacy of current reprocessing procedures and highlighting a specialty-wide challenge, because more than 600,000 ERCPs are completed annually in the United States.[30] New technologies are on the horizon to address the challenge of duodenoscope reprocessing. The proposed solutions include single-use duodeno scopes, and reusable duodenoscopes with detachable distal caps, which may allow more thorough cleaning of the elevator mechanism. The high cost of a single-use duo denoscope is of particular concern, and so it is expected that initially single-use duo denoscopes may be used selectively for patients at particularly high risk for duodenoscope infection. For instance, cholangiocarcinoma has been identified as a risk factor for carbapenem-resistant Enterobacteriaceae transmission during ERCP,[31] supporting the hypothesis that patients with biliary obstruction are at higher risk of infectious adverse events. It is in this high-risk population, with potential incom plete biliary drainage, whereby the single-use duodenoscope may be most beneficial. Cost analysis estimated the per-procedure cost to vary from US$797 to US$1547 for high-volume centers and US$1318 to US$2068 for low-volume centers.[32] As these technologies continue to develop and are adopted by the gastroenterology commu nity, it remains to be seen whether they will be an effective means in reducing duodenoscope-transmitted infections, particularly in high-risk patient groups.

Patients with Cirrhosis

In patients with cirrhosis, the transition from compensated to decompensated cirrhosis occurs at a rate of 4% to 7% per year.[33] Along with the effects of the hyper dynamic circulatory syndrome, decompensated cirrhotics have increased intestinal permeability and abnormal bacterial translocation. In patients with advanced liver dis ease, the portal hypertensive mechanisms described above could theoretically in crease the risk of bacterial translocation. Cirrhotic patients undergoing routine elective endoscopy must be considered differently than cirrhotic patients undergoing endoscopy for variceal bleeding, because the considerations for antibiotic use differ

Current clinical evidence and guidelines do not support antibiotic prophylaxis for cirrhotic patients undergoing elective endoscopy.[13,34] A prospective study enrolled 60 patients who underwent 112 elective endoscopic variceal ligations (EVL).[35] In 2.7% of procedures, blood cultures returned positive after endoscopy, although these were not clinically relevant infections. Seven previous studies with a cumulative num ber of 176 patients and 247 procedures assessed bacteremia after elective EVL with heterogenous results.[36–42] Positive blood cultures ranged from 0% to 25%, with no clinical significance reported. Overall, elective EVL in cirrhotic patients is considered low risk, and antibiotic prophylaxis is not recommended.

In cirrhotic patients presenting with acute GI bleeding, 2 metaanalyses have shown that antibiotic prophylaxis reduced overall mortality and incidence of bacterial infec tions. It is important to emphasize that the infection risk in this setting is not known to be related to the endoscopy itself, but rather to the observation that patients pre senting with variceal bleed have heightened risk for spontaneous bacterial peritonitis and sepsis. The first metaanalysis from 1999 included 5 trials, encompassing 534 pa tients, and showed that short-term antibiotic prophylaxis significantly increased short term survival rate and the number of patients free of infection.[43] An updated Cochrane review from 2011 included 12 trials, encompassing 1241 patients, and antibiotic pro phylaxis was found to have reduced mortality, mortality from bacterial infection, and rates of bacterial infection.[44] In addition, the rates of rebleeding and days of hospital ization were lower. All cirrhotic patients with acute GI bleeding should be administered antibiotic prophylaxis, regardless of whether endoscopy is performed as part of the treatment protocol.

Ceftriaxone is recommended as the first choice for patients with advanced cirrhosis, for those on quinolone prophylaxis, and in hospital settings with a high prevalence of quinolone-resistant bacteremia.[13] Oral quinolones can be used in other patients and as a step down from intravenous (IV) therapy. A short, 7-day course is recommended for prophylaxis.

Peritoneal Dialysis

Peritonitis is a major cause of adverse events in patients receiving continuous ambulatory peritoneal dialysis (CAPD) and the main reason many patients transition to hemodialysis.[45,46] One mechanism of the development of peritonitis is bacterial translocation from the bowel lumen into the peritoneal cavity, which can occur spontaneously, but may also occur during manipulation of the GI tract. Numerous case series have described peritonitis following colonoscopic polypectomy in CAPD patients.[47–52] Two retrospective studies evaluated the risk of peritonitis following colonoscopy, and this ranged from 6.3% to 8.1%.[53,54] In both studies, there were no cases of peritonitis in patients given antibiotic prophylaxis. Correspondingly, the International Society for Peritoneal Dialysis[55] and American Society for Gastrointestinal Endoscopy (ASGE)[13] recommend the use of prophylactic antibiotics to reduce the risk of peritonitis in CAPD patients undergoing lower endoscopy.

In summary, patients undergoing ERCP with expected incomplete biliary drainage and peritoneal dialysis patients requiring colonoscopy are at high risk of postprocedure infection, and antibiotic prophylaxis should be considered. Incomplete biliary drainage is commonly seen in patients with primary sclerosing cholangitis, cholangiocarcinoma, and other hepatobiliary malignancies. There was previous concern for IE in high-risk cardiac patients; however, unless there is a concomitant GI tract infection, antibiotic prophylaxis is not warranted. In addition, cirrhotic patients presenting with variceal bleeding should also receive antibiotics, although the infectious risk in this setting is not likely related to the endoscopy itself. Immunosuppressed patients represent a high-risk group of patients and are discussed in the following section.

SPECIAL POPULATIONS

Immunosuppressed patients are at increased risk for iatrogenic infection. This population of patients includes but is not limited to organ transplant recipients, patients with advanced human immunodeficiency virus (HIV)/AIDS, common variable immunodeficiency syndrome, and hematologic malignancies. There is a paucity of data regarding infectious adverse events related to GI endoscopy in these patient populations. The literature on endoscopy in HIV/AIDS patients has primarily focused on the risk of viral transmission between patients from contaminated endoscopes. To date, there have been no reported cases.[6,56] In this section, patients with hematologic malignancies, which represent a special population at higher risk of iatrogenic infection during GI endoscopy, are the focus.

Bone Marrow Transplant

The most studied group of immunosuppressed patients undergoing endoscopy is the bone marrow transplant (BMT) population. There have been several retrospective studies that have addressed the risk of endoscopy following BMT and the role of prophylactic antibiotics. In this population, the most common indication for endoscopy was for the diagnosis of graft-versus-host disease. Neutropenia and thrombocytopenia were identified as risk factors for adverse events, although the definition of each varied by study. In a retrospective analysis of 67 procedures in BMT recipients, a single patient who did not receive antibiotics developed clinically relevant bacteremia, whereas patients on antibiotics had no adverse events.[57] In a pediatric population undergoing percutaneous endoscopic gastrostomy (PEG) tube insertion after BMT, complications only occurred in patients with neutropenia, despite routine periprocedural cephalexin.[58] In a review of 191 pediatric patients undergoing diagnostic endoscopy following BMT, complications occurred in 13 procedures, 12 of which were GI bleeding. Thrombocytopenia was identified as the only significant risk factor.[59] Limited available data suggest that routine endoscopy in patients after BMT is safe, with neutropenia and thrombocytopenia identified as risk factors for adverse events.

Neutropenia

Neutropenia is most commonly seen in oncology patients following chemotherapy, after immunosuppression in BMT patients, or in advanced hematologic malignancy.

A systematic review from 2015 evaluated 8 studies in which endoscopy for a variety of indications was completed for neutropenic patients.[60] Neutropenia was generally defined as an absolute neutrophil count (ANC) of less than 500 cells/mm^3, and in all studies, patients with febrile neutropenia received antibiotics. Postprocedure fever was reported in up to 15% of patients who did not receive antibiotics before the procedure, although this was not clinically significant.[61]

A retrospective study from 2019 identified 588 patients with cancer who underwent 675 endoscopic procedures in the setting of neutropenia.[62] Most patients had a hematologic malignancy. Neutropenia was defined as an ANC less than 1000 cells/μL. Within 1 week of endoscopy, 4% of patients experienced infectious adverse events. There was no association between ANC level and risk of infectious adverse events. Antibiotics were given in 70% of patients in this study and 91% of patients with severe neutropenia (ANC <200 cells/μL). Propensity score matching found the use of prophylactic antibiotics did not decrease the risk of infectious adverse events.

In summary, limited data are available in the population of immunosuppressed and neutropenic patients. Most data are retrospective and arise from patients with hematologic malignancies. International guidelines are similarly based off of low-quality evidence. The ASGE does not make a recommendation for or against the use of prophylactic antibiotics for routine endoscopy. In patients with an ANC less than 500 cells/μL, the ASGE suggests the decision to use antibiotics should be individualized.[13] In the same population, the British Society of Gastroenterology[21] and European Society of Gastrointestinal Endoscopy[63] guidelines recommend the use of prophylactic antibiotics only in procedures with a high risk of bacteremia, such as sclerotherapy, dilation, and ERCP in an obstructed system.

Routine endoscopy appears safe in BMT patients, with thrombocytopenia and neutropenia identified as risk factors for adverse events. Neutropenic patients have a low risk of adverse events, and prophylactic antibiotics do not appear to change outcomes. Preprocedure antibiotics should be administered for febrile neutropenic patients and neutropenic patients undergoing high-risk procedures.

HIGH-RISK PROCEDURES

Endoscopic procedures with the highest risk of transient bacteremia include esophageal dilation, sclerotherapy of varices, and instrumentation of obstructed bile ducts during ERCP. The rate of bacteremia in esophageal dilation has been estimated at 12% to 22%,[64,65] with rates shown to be higher in malignant strictures.[65]

clerotherapy has reported rates of bacteremia as high as 52%.[66] EVL and instrumen-
ition of obstructed bile ducts were covered earlier in this article. This section focuses
n established as well as emerging procedures with a high risk of infectious adverse
vents.

holangioscopy and Pancreatoscopy

ne mean rate of bacteremia following routine ERCP is 6.4%.[67] In an obstructed sys-
2m, this increases to 18%,[67] and current ASGE guidelines recommend prophylactic
ntibiotics only in patients in whom incomplete biliary drainage is expected.[13] Cholan-
ioscopy presents a different set of risks because procedures are often performed in
1e setting of obstructed systems: biliary strictures, difficult stones, and cholangiocar-
inoma, among other indications. The risk profile is further increased by the longer
uration of cholangioscopic procedures, the use of additional instrumentation within
1e common bile duct, such as electrohydraulic lithotripsy, and the necessity for irri-
ation with water or saline. Fluid irrigation may increase intrabiliary pressures and
1erefore increase the risk of procedure-related bacteremia.[68]

There have been 3 single-center studies on the risk of infectious adverse events
illowing cholangioscopy or pancreatoscopy **(Table 2)**.[69–71] Sethi and colleagues[69]
xamined 4214 ERCPs, 402 of which included cholangioscopy or pancreatoscopy.
ompared with the ERCP-only cohort, patients undergoing cholangioscopy or pan-
reatoscopy had higher rates of adverse events (2.9% vs 7%, odds ratio [OR], 2.50;
5% confidence interval [CI], 1.56–3.89), and significantly higher rates of cholangitis
).2% vs 1%, OR, 4.98; 95% CI, 1.06–19.67). Patients in the other 2 studies underwent
holangioscopy only. In all 3 studies, prophylactic antibiotics were administered peri-
rocedure. Thosani and colleagues[71] identified biliary strictures and patients undergo-
ig intraductal biopsies as higher risk. Furthermore, in all 3 studies, it was postulated
iat complications were secondary to copious intraductal irrigation required during
holangioscopy.

Although limited, the data suggest a high rate of bacteremia (7%–10%) and cholan-
itis (1%–7%) associated with cholangioscopy. Given the indications for cholangio-
copy, generally in patients with an obstructed biliary system requiring increased
itraductal manipulation, higher rates of bacteremia are not unexpected, and prophy-
ictic antibiotics are suggested.

ndoscopic Ultrasound with Tissue Acquisition

ndoscopic ultrasound (EUS) -guided fine-needle aspiration (FNA) and fine-needle bi-
psy (FNB) are common techniques for tissue acquisition of solid and cystic lesions.
Vith advances in abdominal imaging, pancreatic cysts are being identified more

Table 2
Studies examining the risk of infection following cholangioscopy or pancreatoscopy

Study, Year	Type	Total Patients	Outcomes
Sethi et al,[69] 2011	Retrospective	402	Adverse events: 7% Cholangitis: 1%
Othman et al,[70] 2016	Prospective	72	Bacteremia: 10% Cholangitis: 7%
Thosani et al,[71] 2016	Prospective	57	Bacteremia: 9% Cholangitis: 7%

frequently, and EUS FNA is often used to inform diagnosis and management. Despite the increase in endoscopic volume, there remain limited data on infectious complications related to EUS FNA of cystic lesions.

EUS FNA or FNB of solid lesions is considered low risk, and antibiotic prophylaxis is currently not recommended. An early study from 1999 retrospectively evaluated 32 EUS FNA procedures, 10 of which were for cystic lesions.[72] Only 1 infectious complication was noted, which was of a pancreatic tail cyst. There were no complications noted, infectious or otherwise, in EUS FNA of solid lesions. A study involving 355 consecutive patients undergoing EUS FNA of solid pancreatic masses only had 2 patients (0.56%) develop infectious symptoms requiring the use of antibiotics after the procedure.[13] An additional 4 prospective studies comprising more than 700 EUS FNA of solid lesions had rates of bacteremia of up to 6%, but none of which were clinically significant, requiring treatment.[73–76] EUS FNA of solid lesions appears safe with very low rates of bacteremia, and even lower rates of clinically significant infection. EUS FNB is a more recent innovation, but the authors believe that the infection risk should be no different than FNA for solid lesions. Prophylactic antibiotics are not suggested.

Current guidelines recommend antibiotic prophylaxis for EUS FNA of cystic lesions, citing a higher rate of febrile episodes and infectious complications.[21,77] Four studies have reported on the rate of adverse events following EUS FNA of cystic lesions (**Table 3**).[78–81] An early study reported a 10% rate of infectious complications following EUS FNA of pancreatic cystic lesions; however, this has not been consistent with more recent data.[78] In the Guarner-Argente and colleagues[81] study, one-third of patients received antibiotics, and the only clinically significant infection occurred in a patient who received antibiotic prophylaxis. There remain limited data on the use of prophylactic antibiotics in FNA of cystic pancreatic lesions. With the exception of early studies, the infectious complication rate appears low with or without the use of prophylactic antibiotics.

Several case reports have indicated an increased risk of infection following EUS FNA of mediastinal cysts, including life-threatening mediastinitis.[82–87] A prospective study performed EUS FNA in 22 mediastinal cysts with patients receiving prophylactic antibiotics, with no reported adverse events or infectious complications.[88] However, 2 case series reported complications despite the use of preprocedure and postprocedure antibiotics.[85,87] It has been postulated that the protein-rich content of mediastinal

Table 3
Infectious adverse events following endoscopic ultrasound fine-needle aspiration of cystic lesions

Study, Year	Study Type	Total Patients	Prophylactic Antibiotics	Outcomes
Wiersema et al,[78] 1997	Prospective	22	Not specified	Infectious AER: 10%
O'Toole et al,[79] 2001	Prospective	114	66% of patients	AER: 1.2% Infectious AER: None
Lee et al,[80] 2005	Retrospective	651	>90% of patients	AER: 2.2% Infectious AER: 0.15%
Guarner-Argente et al,[81] 2011	Retrospective	266	33% of patients	AP–Infectious AER: 1.14% NAP–Infectious AER: 0.6%

Abbreviations: AER, adverse event rate; AP, antibiotic prophylaxis; NAP, no antibiotic prophylaxis cysts provides a fertile medium for bacterial growth from the oropharynx.[85] Currently, both the ASGE and the European Society of Gastrointestinal Endoscopy guidelines recommend the use of prophylactic antibiotics when sampling mediastinal cysts, with patient selection paramount in the decision-making process.[77,89]

Lumen Apposing Metal Stents

Lumen apposing metal stents (LAMS) have ushered in a new era of therapeutic EUS. Although LAMS were developed to treat pancreatic fluid collections (PFC), several novel applications for LAMS, including choledochoduodenostomy, EUS-guided gallbladder drainage, gastrojejunostomy, and EUS-directed transgastric ERCP, have generated much enthusiasm in the interventional EUS community. Because these techniques remain in the developmental phase, this section focuses on LAMS for PFC treatment.

Initially introduced in 2014, LAMS have now been widely accepted as first-line therapy for drainage of PFCs, including pseudocysts and walled off pancreatic necrosis. Infectious adverse events range from 1% to 10% (**Table 4**).[90–95] In all studies, patients received preprocedure antibiotics, and in most studies, a course of oral postprocedure antibiotics. The retrospective cohort study by Puga and colleagues[94] in 41 patients compared LAMS with LAMS plus double pigtail for PFCs, with an overall infection rate of 10%. The LAMS-alone group had a higher infectious event rate; however, this was not statistically significant. Infections related to LAMS for PFC in both the wire-guided and electrocautery enhanced systems appear low, and the most recent data describe only a 1% rate of infection. For many of these patients, the indication for cyst gastrostomy was infected pancreatic necrosis, and this population would already be maintained on antibiotics.

Overall, current practice favors the use of periprocedural antibiotics during the treatment of PFC, although the data available to guide specific decisions on antibiotic choice and duration are limited. As with ERCP, if there is a likelihood of incomplete drainage after initial LAMS placement (particularly relevant for walled-off necrosis and/or loculated collections), then periprocedural antibiotics are likely of higher importance.

Table 4
Infectious adverse event rate following lumen apposing metal stent placement for pancreatic fluid collections

Study, Year	Study Type	Total Patients	LAMS Type	Outcomes
Shah et al,[90] 2015	Multicenter, prospective	33	Wire guided	Infectious AER: 3%
Rinninella et al,[91] 2015	Multicenter, retrospective	93	Cautery enhanced	Overall AER: 5% Infectious AER: 1%
Sharaiha et al,[92] 2016	Multicenter, retrospective	124	Wire guided	Overall AER: 18.5% Infectious AER: 6%
Yang et al,[93] 2018	Multicenter, retrospective	122	62% Cautery enhanced	Infectious AER: 5.6%
Puga et al,[94] 2018	Retrospective cohort	41	49% Cautery enhanced	Overall AER: 27% Infectious AER: 10%
Kumta et al,[96] 2019	Multicenter, prospective	192	15.6% Cautery enhanced	Overall AER: 7.8% Infectious AER: 1%

Endoscopic Mucosal Resection and Endoscopic Submucosal Dissection

Endoscopic mucosal resection (EMR) and endoscopic submucosal dissection (ESD) are increasingly common techniques used to remove large lesions in the GI tract. In both EMR and ESD, submucosal injection is required to lift the lesion to facilitate removal. In many cases, more than 1 submucosal injection is required, thus creating a theoretic risk of infection, because repeat submucosal injection can introduce bacteria into the submucosal space. In addition, a large defect results after resection, which exposes the tissue to endogenous bacterial flora. Current guidelines from Japan do not support the use of prophylactic antibiotics for EMR or ESD,[97] and this is not addressed in American or European guidelines.

In a prospective study of 38 patients undergoing upper GI EMR, blood cultures were obtained at 10 minutes and 4 hours after procedures.[98] There were 2 positive blood cultures at 10 minutes, and none at 4 hours. In the lower GI tract, a prospective study of 33 patients measured blood cultures at 5 and 30 minutes after the procedure, with 1 positive culture at 30 minutes.[99] The offending organism was coagulase-negative *Staphylococcus* and was determined to be a contaminant. In a large prospective study of 479 patients undergoing colorectal EMR, 1.5% of patients required antibiotics for suspected serositis, defined as abdominal pain and fever without signs of perforation after the procedure.[100] Blood cultures were not measured. In another study of 214 patients undergoing EMR or ESD, half of the patients were randomized to receive prophylactic antibiotics.[101] Nearly 60% of the cases were EMR. Fever was significantly lower in the group that received antibiotics (0.9% vs 8.4%, $P<.05$), and 2 patients had positive blood cultures in the control group, compared with none in the antibiotic group. The study did not differentiate whether the complications were in the EMR or ESD population. In addition, fever was conservatively defined as 37.2°C or greater. The risk of bacteremia and infection following EMR is low, and prophylactic antibiotics are not suggested.

Rates of bacteremia are similarly low in patients undergoing ESD. Three prospective studies measured blood cultures immediately after and at various intervals after ESD. In all studies, the rate of bacteremia was 4%, and in only 1 study, there was a sustained bacteremia.[102–104] In all cases, bacteremia was clinically not significant, and no antibiotics were required.

A known but underreported complication of ESD is post-ESD electrocoagulation syndrome (PEECS). PEECS is characterized by signs and symptoms of peritoneal inflammation without evidence of perforation. Patients present with abdominal pain, fever, and leukocytosis. Treatment is generally conservative with bowel rest, IV antibiotics, and IV fluids. The pathophysiology of PEECS is thought to be related to excessive coagulation causing inflammation, and it is possible that this pathophysiology could increase the risk of infection as well. The rate of PEECS has been reported between 7% and 65%, with large lesion size and longer ESD duration consistently noted as risk factors.[105–108] A recent clinical trial randomized 100 patients undergoing colorectal ESD to receive antibiotics versus no antibiotics. The antibiotic group had a significantly lower incidence of PEECS with only 1 case, compared with 8 cases in the control group. In addition, the antibiotic group had lower rates of abdominal pain and elevated CRP. The use of prophylactic antibiotics may be useful to reduce the rates of PEECS in the ESD population, but further study is required.

In summary, the rates of bacteremia are low in EMR and ESD, and bacteremia is rarely clinically significant. There are not enough data to support prophylactic antibiotics for these procedures.

ercutaneous Endoscopic Gastrostomy

EG tubes provide a short- or long-term nutrition solution for patients who are unable ɔ tolerate an oral diet. PEG tubes are able to deliver a liquid diet or medications. Paents undergoing PEG tube placement are vulnerable to infection because of age, ompromised nutritional status, immunosuppression, and underlying medical comoridities. International guidelines support the use of systemic antibiotics to prevent inections related to PEG placement.[13,21,63]

A Cochrane Collaboration systematic review and metaanalysis evaluated the role of rophylactic systemic antimicrobial drugs to reduce the risk of peristomal infections in atients undergoing PEG tube placement.[109] Twelve trials encompassing 1271 paents were included in the metaanalysis. The pooled analysis included trials that ompared antibiotics to placebo, no intervention, or skin antiseptic and showed onsistent beneficial effects for antibiotic use (OR 0.36; 95% CI 0.26–0.50). These ndings are in keeping with previous systematic reviews.[110,111] Broad-spectrum antiiotics with activity against cutaneous organisms are suggested for PEG tube inserɔn to prevent the rate of peristomal infections.

ndoscopic Sleeve Gastroplasty

ndoscopic sleeve gastroplasty (ESG) is an emerging weight loss option for patients who ave failed medical therapy and are not candidates for surgical intervention. During ESG, astric capacity is reduced by endoscopically placed full-thickness sutures along the reater curve of the stomach. The most common adverse events reported in up to 0% of ESG are postprocedure abdominal pain and bleeding.[112] There is a lack of data n infectious adverse events, and this may be due to a combination of underreporting nd low rates of infectious complications. A review of 1000 consecutive patients at a sin-le center reported a 0.5% rate of fever with no associated bacteremia and 0.4% rate of erigastric collections managed with broad-spectrum antibiotics.[113] A retrospective re-iew of 248 ESG patients across 3 centers had 2 cases of perigastric fluid collections ɛquiring drainage and antibiotics.[114] An additional 3 cases of intraabdominal collections fter the procedure have been described, 2 cases treated with percutaneous drainage nd 1 case with antibiotics.[115–117] A metaanalysis comprising 9 studies and 1542 patients ad a pooled rate of severe adverse events of 1%, which included perigastric fluid collecɔns, pulmonary embolism, pneumoperitoneum, pneumothorax, and bleeding requiring ʾansfusion. Limited available data show a low rate of infectious adverse events related to SG, with perigastric fluid collections the most commonly reported.

n summary, more than 20 million GI endoscopic procedures are completed in the Inited States annually with routine procedures having very low rates of infectious dverse events. ERCP in obstructed biliary systems, endoscopic manipulation of fluid ollections, and sinus/fistula tract formation are high risk for infection, and antibiotic ɾrophylaxis is warranted. Emerging procedures, particularly in the rapidly expanding eld of therapeutic EUS, require further study.

UMMARY

il endoscopy remains a safe and effective means for the diagnosis and management ɨf GI diseases. Endogenous and exogenous factors can increase the risk of infectious dverse events, as described in this article. As endoscopy becomes increasingly ther-ɨpeutic in nature, the need for prophylaxis will continue to be a topic of discussion, ɨnd high-quality studies are necessary. The concurrent concerns of antibiotic resis-ance require judicious and individualized use of antibiotic prophylaxis.

CONFLICTS OF INTEREST

Dr T.M. Berzin is a consultant for Boston Scientific and Fujifilm.

REFERENCES

1. Joseph DA, Meester RGS, Zauber AG, et al. Colorectal cancer screening: esti mated future colonoscopy need and current volume and capacity. Cancer 2016 122(16):2479–86.
2. Al-Awabdy B, Wilcox CM. Use of anesthesia on the rise in gastrointestina endoscopy. World J Gastrointest Endosc 2013;5(1):1.
3. Baltch AL, Buhac I, Agrawal A, et al. Bacteremia after upper gastrointestina endoscopy. Arch Intern Med 1977;137(5):594.
4. Mellow MH, Lewis RJ. Endoscopy-related bacteremia. Arch Intern Med 1976 136(6):667.
5. Shull HJ, Greene BM, Allen SD, et al. Bacteremia with upper gastrointestina endoscopy. Ann Intern Med 1975;83(2):212.
6. Kovaleva J, Peters FTM, van der Mei HC, et al. Transmission of Infection by flex ible gastrointestinal endoscopy and bronchoscopy. Clin Microbiol Rev 2013 26(2):231–54.
7. Rutter CM, Johnson E, Miglioretti DL, et al. Adverse events after screening anc follow-up colonoscopy. Cancer Causes Control 2012;23(2):289–96.
8. Nelson DB. Infectious disease complications of GI endoscopy: part II, exoge nous infections. Gastrointest Endosc 2003;57(6):695–711.
9. Fisher DA, Maple JT, Ben-Menachem T, et al. Complications of colonoscopy Gastrointest Endosc 2011;74(4):745–52.
10. Wilson W, Taubert KA, Gewitz M, et al. Prevention of infective endocarditis. Cir culation 2007;116(15):1736–54.
11. Forner L, Larsen T, Kilian M, et al. Incidence of bacteremia after chewing, tooth brushing and scaling in individuals with periodontal inflammation. J Clin Perio dontol 2006;33(6):401–7.
12. Schlein RA, Kudlick EM, Reindorf CA, et al. Toothbrushing and transient bacter emia in patients undergoing orthodontic treatment. Am J Orthod Dentofac Or thop 1991;99(5):466–72.
13. Khashab MA, Chithadi KV, Acosta RD, et al. Antibiotic prophylaxis for GI endos copy. Gastrointest Endosc 2015;81(1):81–9.
14. Dajani AS, Taubert KA, Wilson W, et al. Prevention of bacterial endocarditis. Cir culation 1997;96(1):358–66.
15. Masci E, Toti G, Mariani A, et al. Complications of diagnostic and therapeutic ERCP: a prospective multicenter study. Am J Gastroenterol 2001;96(2):417–23
16. Ong T-Z, Khor J-L, Selamat D-S, et al. Complications of endoscopic retrograde cholangiography in the post-MRCP era: a tertiary center experience. World J Gastroenterol 2005;11(33):5209–12.
17. Andriulli A, Loperfido S, Napolitano G, et al. Incidence rates of post-ERCP com plications: a systematic survey of prospective studies. Am J Gastroenterol 2007 102(8):1781–8.
18. Williams EJ, Taylor S, Fairclough P, et al. Risk factors for complication following ERCP; results of a large-scale, prospective multicenter study. Endoscopy 2007 39(9):793–801.
19. Ismail S, Kylänpää L, Mustonen H, et al. Risk factors for complications of ERCP in primary sclerosing cholangitis. Endoscopy 2012;44(12):1133–8.

20. Bangarulingam SY, Gossard AA, Petersen BT, et al. Complications of endoscopic retrograde cholangiopancreatography in primary sclerosing cholangitis. Am J Gastroenterol 2009;104(4):855–60.
21. Allison MC, Sandoe JAT, Tighe R, et al. Antibiotic prophylaxis in gastrointestinal endoscopy. Gut 2009;58(6):869–80.
22. Manes G, Paspatis G, Aabakken L, et al. Endoscopic management of common bile duct stones: European Society of Gastrointestinal Endoscopy (ESGE) guideline. Endoscopy 2019;51(05):472–91.
23. Harris A, Chong H, Chan A, et al. Meta-analysis of antibiotic prophylaxis in endoscopic retrograde cholangiopancreatography (ERCP). Endoscopy 1999; 31(9):718–24.
24. Bai Y, Gao F, Gao J, et al. Prophylactic antibiotics cannot prevent endoscopic retrograde cholangiopancreatography-induced cholangitis. Pancreas 2009; 38(2):126–30.
25. Brand M, Bizos D, O'Farrell PJ. Antibiotic prophylaxis for patients undergoing elective endoscopic retrograde cholangiopancreatography. Cochrane Database Syst Rev 2010;(10):CD007345.
26. Cotton PB, Connor P, Rawls E, et al. Infection after ERCP, and antibiotic prophylaxis: a sequential quality-improvement approach over 11 years. Gastrointest Endosc 2008;67(3):471–5.
27. Rahman MR, Perisetti A, Coman R, et al. Duodenoscope-associated infections: update on an emerging problem. Dig Dis Sci 2019;64(6):1409–18.
28. Rauwers AW, Voor in 't holt AF, Buijs JG, et al. High prevalence rate of digestive tract bacteria in duodenoscopes: a nationwide study. Gut 2018;67(9):1637–45.
29. The FDA continues to remind facilities of the importance of following duodenoscope reprocessing instructions: FDA safety communication. US Food and Drug Administration. Available at: https://www.fda.gov/medical-devices/safety-communications/fda-continues-remind-facilities-importance-following-duodeno scope-reprocessing-instructions-fda. Accessed August 21, 2019.
30. Petersen BT, Cohen J, Hambrick RD, et al. Multisociety guideline on reprocessing flexible GI endoscopes: 2016 update. Gastrointest Endosc 2017;85(2): 282–94.e1.
31. Kim S, Russell D, Mohamadnejad M, et al. Risk factors associated with the transmission of carbapenem-resistant Enterobacteriaceae via contaminated duodenoscopes. Gastrointest Endosc 2016;83(6):1121–9.
32. Bang JY, Sutton B, Hawes R, Varadarajulu S. Concept of disposable duodenoscope: at what cost? Gut 2019;68:1915–7.
33. D'Amico G, Garcia-Tsao G, Pagliaro L. Natural history and prognostic indicators of survival in cirrhosis: a systematic review of 118 studies. J Hepatol 2006;44(1): 217–31.
34. Angeli P, Bernardi M, Villanueva C, et al. EASL Clinical Practice Guidelines for the management of patients with decompensated cirrhosis. J Hepatol 2018; 69(2):406–60.
35. Maimone S, Saffioti F, Filomia R, et al. Elective endoscopic variceal ligation is not a risk factor for bacterial infection in patients with liver cirrhosis. Dig Liver Dis 2018;50(4):366–9.
36. Tseng CC, Green RM, Burke SK, et al. Bacteremia after endoscopic band ligation of esophageal varices. Gastrointest Endosc 1992;38(3):336–7.
37. Berner JS, Gaing AA, Sharma R, et al. Sequelae after esophageal variceal ligation and sclerotherapy: a prospective randomized study. Am J Gastroenterol 1994;89(6):852–8.

38. Kulkarni SG, Parikh SS, Dhawan PS, et al. High frequency of bacteremia with endoscopic treatment of esophageal varices in advanced cirrhosis. Indian J Gastroenterol 1999;18(4):143–5.

39. Lin OS, Wu SS, Chen YY, et al. Bacterial peritonitis after elective endoscopic variceal ligation: a prospective study. Am J Gastroenterol 2000;95(1):214–7.

40. Maulaz EB, de Mattos AA, Pereira-Lima J, et al. Bacteremia in cirrhotic patients submitted to endoscopic band ligation of esophageal varices. Arq Gastroenterol 2003;40(3):166–72.

41. Bonilha DQ, Correia LM, Monaghan M, et al. Prospective study of bacteremia rate after elective band ligation and sclerotherapy with cyanoacrylate for esophageal varices in patients with advanced liver disease. Arq Gastroenterol 2011; 48(4):248–51.

42. Zuckerman MJ, Jia Y, Hernandez JA, et al. A prospective randomized study on the risk of bacteremia in banding versus sclerotherapy of esophageal varices. Front Med 2016;3:16.

43. Bernard B, Grangé J-D, Khac EN, et al. Antibiotic prophylaxis for the prevention of bacterial infections in cirrhotic patients with gastrointestinal bleeding: a meta-analysis. Hepatology 1999;29(6):1655–61.

44. Chavez-Tapia NC, Barrientos-Gutierrez T, Tellez-Avila F, et al. Meta-analysis: antibiotic prophylaxis for cirrhotic patients with upper gastrointestinal bleeding - an updated Cochrane review. Aliment Pharmacol Ther 2011;34(5):509–18.

45. Holley JL, Praino BM. Complications of peritoneal dialysis: diagnosis and management. Semin Dial 1990;3(4):245–8.

46. Stablein DM, Nolph KD, Lindblad AS. Timing and characteristics of multiple peritonitis episodes: a report of the National CAPD Registry. Am J Kidney Dis 1989;14(1):44–9.

47. Verger C, Danne O, Vuillemin F. Colonoscopy and continuous ambulatory peritoneal dialysis. Gastrointest Endosc 1987;33(4):334–5.

48. Petersen JH, Weesner RE, Giannella RA. Escherichia coli peritonitis after left-sided colonoscopy in a patient on continuous ambulatory peritoneal dialysis. Am J Gastroenterol 1987;82(2):171–2.

49. Suh H, Wadhwa NK, Cabralda T, et al. Endogenous peritonitis and related outcome in peritoneal dialysis patients. Adv Perit Dial 1996;12:192–5.

50. Yip T, Tse KC, Lam MF, et al. Risks and outcomes of peritonitis after flexible colonoscopy in CAPD patients. Perit Dial Int 2007;27(5):560–4.

51. Lin Y-C, Lin W-P, Huang J-Y, et al. Polymicrobial peritonitis following colonoscopic polypectomy in a peritoneal dialysis patient. Intern Med 2012;51(14): 1841–3.

52. Gould AL, Chahla E, Hachem C. Peritonitis following endoscopy in a patient on peritoneal dialysis with a discussion of current recommendations on antibiotic prophylaxis. Case Rep Gastroenterol 2015;9(3):302–6.

53. Yip T, Tse KC, Lam MF, et al. Risks and outcomes of peritonitis after flexible colonoscopy in CAPD patients. Perit Dial Int 2007;27(5):560–4.

54. Wu H-H, Li I-J, Weng C-H, et al. Prophylactic antibiotics for endoscopy-associated peritonitis in peritoneal dialysis patients. PLoS One 2013;8(8): e71532.

55. Li PK-T, Szeto CC, Piraino B, et al. ISPD peritonitis recommendations: 2016 update on prevention and treatment. Perit Dial Int 2016;36(5):481–508.

56. Calderwood AH, Day LW, Muthusamy VR, et al. ASGE guideline for infection control during GI endoscopy. Gastrointest Endosc 2018;87(5):1167–79.

57. Kaw M, Przepiorka D, Sekas G. Infectious complications of endoscopic procedures in bone marrow transplant recipients. Dig Dis Sci 1993;38(1):71–4.

58. Kaur S, Ceballos C, Bao R, et al. Percutaneous endoscopic gastrostomy tubes
in pediatric bone marrow transplant patients. J Pediatr Gastroenterol Nutr 2013;
56(3):300–3.

59. Khan K, Schwarzenberg SJ, Sharp H, et al. Diagnostic endoscopy in children
after hematopoietic stem cell transplantation. Gastrointest Endosc 2006;64(3):
379–85.

60. Tong MC, Tadros M, Vaziri H. Endoscopy in neutropenic and/or thrombocyto-
penic patients. World J Gastroenterol 2015;21(46):13166–76.

61. Gorschlüter M, Schmitz V, Mey U, et al. Endoscopy in patients with acute
leukaemia after intensive chemotherapy. Leuk Res 2008;32(10):1510–7.

62. Abu-Sbeih H, Ali FS, Coronel E, et al. Safety of endoscopy in cancer patients
with thrombocytopenia and neutropenia. Gastrointest Endosc 2019;89(5):
937–49.e2.

63. Rey JR, Axon A, Budzynska A, et al. Guidelines of the European Society of
Gastrointestinal Endoscopy (E.S.G.E.) antibiotic prophylaxis for gastrointestinal
endoscopy. European Society of Gastrointestinal Endoscopy. Endoscopy 1998;
30(3):318–24.

64. Zuccaro G, Richter JE, Rice TW, et al. Viridans streptococcal bacteremia after
esophageal stricture dilation. Gastrointest Endosc 1998;48(6):568–73.

65. Nelson DB, Sanderson SJ, Azar MM. Bacteremia with esophageal dilation. Gastrointest Endosc 1998;48(6):563–7.

66. Cohen LB, Korsten MA, Scherl EJ, et al. Bacteremia after endoscopic injection
sclerosis. Gastrointest Endosc 1983;29(3):198–200.

67. Nelson DB. Infectious disease complications of GI endoscopy: part I, endogenous infections. Gastrointest Endosc 2003;57(4):546–56.

68. Lau WY, Fan ST, Yip WC, et al. Optimal irrigation pressures in operative choledochoscopy. Aust N Z J Surg 1988;58(1):63–6.

69. Sethi A, Chen YK, Austin GL, et al. ERCP with cholangiopancreatoscopy may be
associated with higher rates of complications than ERCP alone: a single-center
experience. Gastrointest Endosc 2011;73(2):251–6.

70. Othman MO, Guerrero R, Elhanafi S, et al. A prospective study of the risk of
bacteremia in directed cholangioscopic examination of the common bile duct.
Gastrointest Endosc 2016;83(1):151–7.

71. Thosani N, Zubarik R, Kochar R, et al. Prospective evaluation of bacteremia
rates and infectious complications among patients undergoing single-operator
choledochoscopy during ERCP. Endoscopy 2016;48(05):424–31.

72. Williams DB, Sahai AV, Aabakken L, et al. Endoscopic ultrasound guided fine
needle aspiration biopsy: a large single centre experience. Gut 1999;44(5):
720–6.

73. Levy MJ, Norton ID, Wiersema MJ, et al. Prospective risk assessment of bacteremia and other infectious complications in patients undergoing EUS-guided
FNA. Gastrointest Endosc 2003;57(6):672–8.

74. Levy MJ, Norton ID, Clain JE, et al. Prospective study of bacteremia and complications with EUS FNA of rectal and perirectal lesions. Clin Gastroenterol Hepatol 2007;5(6):684–9.

75. Janssen J, König K, Knop-Hammad V, et al. Frequency of bacteremia after
linear EUS of the upper GI tract with and without FNA. Gastrointest Endosc
2004;59(3):339–44.

76. Barawi M, Gottlieb K, Cunha B, et al. A prospective evaluation of the incidenc of bacteremia associated with EUS-guided fine-needle aspiration. Gastrointe Endosc 2001;53(2):189–92.

77. Early DS, Acosta RD, Chandrasekhara V, et al. Adverse events associated wi EUS and EUS with FNA. Gastrointest Endosc 2013;77(6):839–43.

78. Wiersema MJ, Vilmann P, Giovannini M, et al. Endosonography-guided fin needle aspiration biopsy: diagnostic accuracy and complication assessmer Gastroenterology 1997;112(4):1087–95.

79. O'Toole D, Palazzo L, Arotçarena R, et al. Assessment of complications of EU' guided fine-needle aspiration. Gastrointest Endosc 2001;53(4):470–4.

80. Lee LS, Saltzman JR, Bounds BC, et al. EUS-guided fine needle aspiration pancreatic cysts: a retrospective analysis of complications and their predictor Clin Gastroenterol Hepatol 2005;3(3):231–6.

81. Guarner-Argente C, Shah P, Buchner A, et al. Use of antimicrobials for EU: guided FNA of pancreatic cysts: a retrospective, comparative analysis. Gastr intest Endosc 2011;74(1):81–6.

82. Ryan AG, Zamvar V, Roberts SA. Iatrogenic candidal infection of a mediastin foregut cyst following endoscopic ultrasound-guided fine-needle aspiratio Endoscopy 2002;34(10):838–9.

83. Aerts JGJV, Kloover J, Los J, et al. EUS-FNA of enlarged necrotic lymph node may cause infectious mediastinitis. J Thorac Oncol 2008;3(10):1191–3.

84. Iwashita T, Yasuda I, Uemura S, et al. Infected mediastinal cyst following end scopic ultrasonography-guided fine-needle aspiration with rupture into th esophagus. Dig Endosc 2012;24(5):386.

85. Valli PV, Gubler C, Bauerfeind P. Severe infectious complications after end scopic ultrasound-guided fine needle aspiration of suspected mediastinal dup cation cysts: a case series. Inflamm Intest Dis 2017;1(4):165–71.

86. Annema J, Veseliç M, Versteegh M, et al. Mediastinitis caused by EUS-FNA of bronchogenic cyst. Endoscopy 2003;35(09):791–3.

87. Diehl DL, Cheruvattath R, Facktor MA, et al. Infection after endoscop ultrasound-guided aspiration of mediastinal cysts. Interact Cardiovasc Thora Surg 2010;10(2):338–40.

88. Fazel A, Moezardalan K, Varadarajulu S, et al. The utility and the safety of EU: guided FNA in the evaluation of duplication cysts. Gastrointest Endosc 200. 62(4):575–80.

89. Polkowski M, Larghi A, Weynand B, et al. Learning, techniques, and complica tions of endoscopic ultrasound (EUS)-guided sampling in gastroenterology: E ropean Society of Gastrointestinal Endoscopy (ESGE) Technical Guidelin Endoscopy 2012;44(02):190–206.

90. Shah RJ, Shah JN, Waxman I, et al. Safety and efficacy of endoscop ultrasound-guided drainage of pancreatic fluid collections with lumen apposing covered self-expanding metal stents. Clin Gastroenterol Hepat 2015;13(4):747–52.

91. Rinninella E, Kunda R, Dollhopf M, et al. EUS-guided drainage of pancreat fluid collections using a novel lumen-apposing metal stent on a electrocautery-enhanced delivery system: a large retrospective study (wit video). Gastrointest Endosc 2015;82(6):1039–46.

92. Sharaiha RZ, Tyberg A, Khashab MA, et al. Endoscopic therapy with lumen apposing metal stents is safe and effective for patients with pancreat walled-off necrosis. Clin Gastroenterol Hepatol 2016;14(12):1797–803.

93. Yang D, Perbtani Y, Mramba L, et al. Safety and rate of delayed adverse events with lumen-apposing metal stents (LAMS) for pancreatic fluid collections: a multicenter study. Endosc Int Open 2018;06(10):E1267–75.

94. Puga M, Consiglieri C, Busquets J, et al. Safety of lumen-apposing stent with or without coaxial plastic stent for endoscopic ultrasound-guided drainage of pancreatic fluid collections: a retrospective study. Endoscopy 2018;50(10):1022–6.

95. Kumta NA, Tyberg A, Bhagat VH, et al. EUS-guided drainage of pancreatic fluid collections using lumen apposing metal stents: an international, multicenter experience. Dig Liver Dis 2019;51(11):1557–61.

96. Kumta NA, Tyberg A, Bhagat VH, et al. EUS-guided drainage of pancreatic fluid collections using lumen apposing metal stents: an international, multicenter experience. Dig Liver Dis 2019;51(11):1557–61.

97. Tanaka S, Kashida H, Saito Y, et al. JGES guidelines for colorectal endoscopic submucosal dissection/endoscopic mucosal resection. Dig Endosc 2015;27(4):417–34.

98. Lee T-H, Hsueh P-R, Yeh W-C, et al. Low frequency of bacteremia after endoscopic mucosal resection. Gastrointest Endosc 2000;52(2):223–5.

99. Min B-H, Chang DK, Kim DU, et al. Low frequency of bacteremia after an endoscopic resection for large colorectal tumors in spite of extensive submucosal exposure. Gastrointest Endosc 2008;68(1):105–10.

100. Moss A, Bourke MJ, Williams SJ, et al. Endoscopic mucosal resection outcomes and prediction of submucosal cancer from advanced colonic mucosal neoplasia. Gastroenterology 2011;140(7):1909–18.

101. Zhang Q-S, Han B, Xu J-H, et al. Antimicrobial prophylaxis in patients with colorectal lesions undergoing endoscopic resection. World J Gastroenterol 2015;21(15):4715–21.

102. Kato M, Kaise M, Obata T, et al. Bacteremia and endotoxemia after endoscopic submucosal dissection for gastric neoplasia: pilot study. Gastric Cancer 2012;15(1):15–20.

103. Kawata N, Tanaka M, Kakushima N, et al. The low incidence of bacteremia after esophageal endoscopic submucosal dissection (ESD) obviates the need for prophylactic antibiotics in esophageal ESD. Surg Endosc 2016;30(11):5084–90.

104. Itaba S, Iboshi Y, Nakamura K, et al. Low-frequency of bacteremia after endoscopic submucosal dissection of the stomach. Dig Endosc 2011;23(1):69–72.

105. Qi Z-P, Shi Q, Liu J-Z, et al. Efficacy and safety of endoscopic submucosal dissection for submucosal tumors of the colon and rectum. Gastrointest Endosc 2018;87(2):540–8.e1.

106. Jung D, Youn Y, Jahng J, et al. Risk of electrocoagulation syndrome after endoscopic submucosal dissection in the colon and rectum. Endoscopy 2013;45(09):714–7.

107. Arimoto J, Higurashi T, Kato S, et al. Risk factors for post-colorectal endoscopic submucosal dissection (ESD) coagulation syndrome: a multicenter, prospective, observational study. Endosc Int Open 2018;06(03):E342–9.

108. Ma DW, Youn YH, Jung DH, et al. Risk factors of electrocoagulation syndrome after esophageal endoscopic submucosal dissection. World J Gastroenterol 2018;24(10):1144–51.

109. Lipp A, Lusardi G. Systemic antimicrobial prophylaxis for percutaneous endoscopic gastrostomy. In: Lipp A, editor. Cochrane database of systematic reviews. Chichester (United Kingdom): John Wiley & Sons, Ltd; 2013:CD005571.

110. Jafri NS, Mahid SS, Minor KS, et al. Meta-analysis: antibiotic prophylaxis to prevent peristomal infection following percutaneous endoscopic gastrostomy. Aliment Pharmacol Ther 2007;25(6):647–56.
111. Sharma VK, Howden CW. Meta-analysis of randomized, controlled trials of antibiotic prophylaxis before percutaneous endoscopic gastrostomy. Am J Gastroenterol 2000;95(11):3133–6.
112. Madruga-Neto AC, Bernardo WM, de Moura DTH, et al. The effectiveness of endoscopic gastroplasty for obesity treatment according to FDA thresholds: systematic review and meta-analysis based on randomized controlled trials. Obes Surg 2018;28(9):2932–40.
113. Alqahtani A, Al-Darwish A, Mahmoud AE, et al. Short-term outcomes of endoscopic sleeve gastroplasty in 1000 consecutive patients. Gastrointest Endosc 2019;89(6):1132–8.
114. Lopez-Nava G, Sharaiha RZ, Vargas EJ, et al. Endoscopic sleeve gastroplasty for obesity: a multicenter study of 248 patients with 24 months follow-up. Obes Surg 2017;27(10):2649–55.
115. Sharaiha RZ, Kumta NA, Saumoy M, et al. Endoscopic sleeve gastroplasty significantly reduces body mass index and metabolic complications in obese patients. Clin Gastroenterol Hepatol 2017;15(4):504–10.
116. Abu Dayyeh BK, Acosta A, Camilleri M, et al. Endoscopic sleeve gastroplasty alters gastric physiology and induces loss of body weight in obese individuals. Clin Gastroenterol Hepatol 2017;15(1):37–43.e1.
117. Barola S, Agnihotri A, Khashab M, et al. Perigastric fluid collection after endoscopic sleeve gastroplasty. Endoscopy 2016;48(S 01):E340–1.

Society Guidelines—Where Is the Consensus?

David S. Vitale, MD[a,b], Karl K. Kwok, MD[c], Quin Y. Liu, MD[d],*

KEYWORDS

- Duodenoscope • Infection • Reprocessing • Society guidelines • FDA • CDC

KEY POINTS

- Multiple societies have published duodenoscope reprocessing guidelines to minimize infection risk via duodenoscope transmission.
- Although professional societies broadly have similar guidelines, there are differences among the national and international societies.
- Several guidelines advise considering further steps beyond duodenoscope manufacturers' recommended reprocessing instructions.
- The single most important intervention, emphasized across multiple guidelines, is thorough manual brushing.

INTRODUCTION

Endoscopic retrograde cholangiopancreatography (ERCP) is a high-volume gastrointestinal (GI) procedure in the United States.[1,2] As with any GI endoscopic procedure, pathogen transmission has become a more scrutinized, studied, and recognized risk factor.[3] Contamination and pathogen transmissions via duodenoscopes are of particular concern, given reported post-ERCP infection rates of up to 2% to 4%.[4]

Previously, endoscope infections were attributed to improper reprocessing procedures or handling of the equipment.[4,5] Since 2008, however, there has been a marked increase in endoscope-related infection transmission reported in the United States and Europe, commonly with multidrug-resistant organisms.[1,6,7] Of concern, only a

[a] Division of Gastroenterology, Hepatology and Nutrition, Cincinnati Children's Hospital Medical Center, 3333 Burnet Avenue, Cincinnati, OH, 45229; [b] Department of Pediatrics, University of Cincinnati College of Medicine, 3230 Eden Avenue, Cincinnati, OH, 45267, USA; [c] Southern California Kaiser Permanente Medical Group, 1526 North Edgemont Street, 7th floor, Los Angeles, CA 90027, USA; [d] Department of Medicine and Pediatrics, Digestive Disease Center, Cedars-Sinai Medical Center/David Geffen School of Medicine at UCLA, 8700 Beverly Blvd, Suite 7700, South Tower, Los Angeles, CA 90048, USA
* Corresponding author.
E-mail address: Quin.Liu@cshs.org
Twitter: GI_Guy (K.K.K.)

Gastrointest Endoscopy Clin N Am 30 (2020) 763–779
https://doi.org/10.1016/j.giec.2020.06.008
1052-5157/20/© 2020 Elsevier Inc. All rights reserved.
giendo.theclinics.com

minority of the cases were attributed to inadequate cleaning or storage, while in most cases investigators were not able to identify a cause.

Beginning in 2012, large outbreaks of infectious complications associated with the ERCP procedure became increasingly frequent in the United States. The Olympus Corporation notified the Food and Drug Administration (FDA) of its concerns and the FDA issued a safety advisory in February 2015.[8] By March 2015, Olympus notified health care professionals of new reprocessing instructions for the company's model TJF-Q180V duodenoscope.[9] Furthermore, the FDA published guidance for reprocessing of medical devices in March 2015, as well as issuing a safety communication in August 2015, with specific focus on enhanced duodenoscope reprocessing.[10,11]

As the role of the duodenoscope in the transmission of infection became better recognized, specific guidelines were published and modified by the FDA and multiple gastroenterology societies in the United States and abroad. Guidelines for duodenoscope sampling and culturing have been cosponsored by the Centers for Disease Control and Prevention (CDC) and FDA.[12] A multisociety guidelines was published with support from the American Society for Gastrointestinal Endoscopy (ASGE), American Gastroenterological Association (AGA), American College of Gastroenterology (ACG), and Society of Gastroenterology Nurses and Associates (SGNA), among other various societies.[2] The SGNA published a separate guideline in 2016 and the most recent iteration in December 2018.[13,14] In addition, many international guidelines have been published, including from British, Canadian, European, Chinese, and Australian societies. This article summarizes national and international guidelines and compares and contrasts the various recommendations related to duodenoscope reprocessing (**Table 1**).

GUIDELINES
Domestic Guidelines

United States – Food and Drug Administration (FDA) and Centers for Disease Control and Prevention (CDC)

The US FDA published a 40-page document in March 2015 outlining recommendations for reprocessing of any reusable medical devices.[10–12] The stated purpose of the document was to guide medical device manufacturers in creating and validating reprocessing instructions for safe use of these reusable devices. The guideline recommends design of reusable devices to facilitate effective and easy cleaning, along with facilitation of any required disinfection or sterilization. The outlined process includes point-of-use processing with prompt initial treatment and removal of contaminants followed by thorough cleaning, followed by low-level disinfection, intermediate-level disinfection, or high-level disinfection (HLD) and/or sterilization. Consistent reprocessing instructions across manufacturer product lines is encouraged. Six criteria were designated for reprocessing instructions: (1) labeling should reflect the intended use of the device; (2) reprocessing instructions for reusable devices should advise users to thoroughly clean the device; (3) reprocessing instructions should indicate the appropriate microbicidal process for the device; (4) reprocessing instructions should be technically feasible and include only devices and accessories that are legally marketed; (5) reprocessing instructions should be comprehensive; and (6) reprocessing instructions should be understandable. There is no specific focus or instruction for reprocessing of flexible endoscopes within the document.

Despite adequate reprocessing technique, some duodenoscopes may have persistent microbial contamination. The FDA introduced the *Supplemental Measures to Enhance Duodenoscope Reprocessing: FDA Safety Communication*[10] in August

Society guidelines and recommendations

Society/Agency	Manual Cleaning	Automated Endoscope Reprocessor	Additional High-Level Disinfection Cycle	Duodenoscope Culturing	Duodenoscope Sterilization	Adenosine Triphosphate Testing	Storage Time Prior to Reprocessing	Loupe Magnification or Borescope	Reprocessing Staff	Disposable Duodenoscope Components
FDA and CDC	Yes—must perform prior to AER	Utilize per manufacturer protocol	Consider as additional reprocessing step.	Consider as additional reprocessing step.	Consider as additional reprocessing step.	Advises not to use ATP testing	NR	NR	Appropriately trained staff	Yes—recommends but understands technology is under development
Multisociety—ASGE/AGA/ACG	Yes—must perform prior to AER	• Consider daily (if not more frequently) testing of HLD fluid. • Manual cleaning still required even if AER labeled as not requiring manual cleaning	Consider as additional reprocessing step (defers to FDA recommendations).	Consider as additional reprocessing step (defers to FDA recommendations).	Consider as additional reprocessing step (defers to FDA recommendations).	NR	NR. Does cite studies ranging from 5–21 d	NR	Annual competency assessment, at introduction of new technology, or if breach identified	NR

(continued on next page)

Table 1
(continued)

Society/ Agency	Manual Cleaning	Automated Endoscope Reprocessor	Additional High-Level Disinfection Cycle	Duode- noscope Culturing	Duode- noscope Sterilization	Aden- osine Tripho- sphate Testing	Storage Time Prior to Repro- cessing	Loupe Magnification or Borescope	Reproc- essing Staff	Dispo- sable Duode- noscope Comp- onents
SGNA	Yes—must perform prior to AER	Test HLD per manufacturer instruction.	Consider as additional reprocessing step (defers to FDA recomm- endations).	Consider as additional reprocessing step (defers to FDA recomm- endations).	Consider as additional reprocessing step (defers to FDA recomm- endations).	NR	7-d interval	Use borescope, if available, for channel inspection.	No temporary staff	NR
ESGE	Yes—must perform prior to AER	Routinely test according to EN ISO 15883.	NR	Culture 25% of duode- noscopes every 3 mo (all duode- noscope will be cultured yearly).	NR	• No recomm- endation • Discusses use to assess duode- noscope cleaning	NR	Use magnifying glass to visually inspect duode- noscope distal- end components.	Only utilize specifically trained staff.	NR

GESA	Yes—must perform prior to AER	NR	• AER should not replace manual cleaning. • AER surveillance cultures Q4 wks	NR	• Elevator scopes tested every 4 wk • All other endoscopes tested every 3 mo	NR	• NR • Discusses use to assess duodenoscope cleaning	• NR • Elevator scopes to be "monitored" every 4 wk. • All other endoscopes "monitored" every 3 mo	• One person should perform full manual cleaning of an endoscope. • If change of shift occurs prior to completion of endoscope reprocessing, the process should be redone. — NR
PHAC	Yes—must perform prior to AER	NR	AER should not replace manual cleaning	NR	No routine culture unless outbreak suspected or confirmed	NR	NR	7-d interval	Utilize sufficiently trained staff. — NR

(continued on next page)

Table 1
(continued)

Society/ Agency	Manual Cleaning	Automated Endoscope Reprocessor	Additional High-Level Disinfection Cycle	Duodenoscope Culturing	Duodenoscope Sterilization	Adenosine Triphosphate Testing	Storage Time Prior to Reprocessing	Loupe Magnification or Borescope	Reprocessing Staff	Disposable Duodenoscope Components
BSG	Yes—must perform prior to AER	• Weekly testing of AER rinse water • Quarterly testing for *P aeruginosa* and mycobacteria	NR	NR	NR	NR	72 h–31 d depending on drying cabinet manufacturer	NR	Annual competency evaluation	Dismantle disposable parts if applicable.
CSDE	Yes—must perform prior to AER	Should be available in advanced endoscopy center "if conditions allow"	NR	Culture every 3 mo.	NR	NR	NR	NR	Regular competency assessment	NR
WEO	Yes—must perform prior to AER	• Perform if resources allow. • Test water periodically.	NR	Randomly test at "routine intervals."	NR	NR	NR	NR	Staff training and monitoring/auditing	NR

| WGO | Yes—must perform prior to AER | • Use AER with submicron filters. • Culture AER at intervals appropriate to local conditions. | • NR • Cites no additional protection against contamination | Monthly surveillance cultures | • NR • Cites no additional protection against contamination | NR | NR | NR | Have "dedicated staff" to reprocess. | NR |

Abbreviations: ACG, American College of Gastroenterology; AER, automated endoscope reprocessor; AGA, American Gastroenterological Association; ASGE, American Society of Gastrointestinal Endoscopy; ATP, Adenosine Triphosphate; BSG, British Society of Gastroenterology; CDC, Centers for Disease Control and Prevention; CSDE, Chinese Society of Digestive Endoscopy; d, day; EN ISO, European Union International Organization for Standardization; FDA, Food and Drug Administration; GESA, Gastroenterological Society of Australia; h, hours; HLD, high level disinfection; mo, month; NR, no recommendation; P aeruginosa, pseudomonas aeruginosa; PHAC, Public Health Agency of Canada; SGNA, Society of Gastroenterology Nurses and Associates; q4 wks, every 4 weeks; WEO, World Endoscopy Organization.

2015. This document outlined supplemental considerations in addition to manufacturers' reprocessing instructions for facilities using duodenoscopes. The guideline supports carefully following manufacturers' instructions for reprocessing and furthermore recommends implementing facility-driven comprehensive quality control programs for duodenoscope reprocessing. The supplemental measures for consideration include ethylene oxide (EtO) sterilization, use of a liquid chemical sterilant processing system, and repeat HLD and microbiological testing. According to the FDA, HLD refers to "a lethal process utilizing sterilant under less than sterilizing conditions. The process kills all forms of microbial life except for large numbers of bacterial spores."[11] The FDA emphasizes that when using any of their suggested supplemental reprocessing measures, prior meticulous manual cleaning and HLD is absolutely essential. The multisociety and SGNA guidelines summarized provide more specific detail regarding these processes.

Within the supplemental processing statement, the FDA recommends sterilization also should be used when possible. Although the guidance suggests EtO gas sterilization after cleaning and HLD be considered, it ultimately recommends following manufacturer instructions regarding use of EtO gas during reprocessing. This sterilization is costly, may prematurely degrade the flexible endoscope, and possibly is toxic to reprocessing personnel and patients if residual EtO is left on the duodenoscope.

Liquid chemical sterilant also should be considered. It is used within a processing device system that utilizes a chemical solution to destroy viable microbial life. Highly purified (not sterile) water then is used to rinse the duodenoscope, although this potentially may result in microbial exposure. Again, this must be used in conjunction with excellent manual cleaning and HLD, and only FDA-cleared processing systems should be used.

The FDA notes that some facilities have implemented a repeat HLD process, using either automated endoscope reprocessors (AERs) or manual HLD, which both are acceptable. Detailed manual cleaning still is required prior to HLD when using this repeat technique.

The additional step of microbiologic culturing the channels and the distal end of the duodenoscopes also is advised if institutionally feasible. There are several options for culturing, including culture after each reprocessing with quarantine until culture result is known, or culturing at fixed intervals for surveillance. The FDA statement, while noting limitations, supports a March 2015 protocol published by the CDC for duodenoscope sampling and culturing, which has since been updated in February 2018 by a working group from the FDA, CDC and the American Society for Microbiology.[12] The 57-page document, *Duodenoscope Surveillance Sampling & Culturing: Reducing the Risks of Infection*, outlines protocols for "surveillance sampling and culturing of reprocessed duodenoscopes intended as a quality control measure of the adequacy of processing." The protocol designs are principally to identify concerning organisms, rather than all potential microbes that could contaminate a duodenoscope. Individual facilities are advised to establish microbial cutoff limits for organisms. The protocols organized into sections that outline materials and methods, and 4 different methods for culturing samples. Two appendices are included, which suggest flush volumes for different channel sizes and include photographs of the sampling process and equipment. The protocol emphasizes that sampling and culturing is optional for health care facilities, except in areas otherwise regulated by state or local policies.

Briefly, the process includes obtaining samples from the instrument channel, elevator recess, and elevator wire channel when it can be accessed. Appropriate personal protection equipment and standard precautions should be followed when obtaining samples. Duodenoscopes never should be taken off site for purpose of ampling and culturing. The sampling should be conducted by appropriately trained taff well versed in handling duodenoscopes, although there are no existing external roficiency testing programs to assure sampling and culturing is adequate or profi-ent. The protocol specifies detailed recommendations for all materials required, etailed methods for obtaining samples, and multiple methods for the culturing rocess.

Other considerations include emphasizing meticulous manual brushing of the levator mechanism and surrounding recesses, even when an AER is used. The levator should be raised and lowered during cleaning to facilitate brushing both des. A quality control program should be implemented at facilities with duodeno-cope reprocessing to include written procedures, monitored training, and other qual-y monitors.

In August 2019, the FDA released a safety communication, *The FDA is Recom-nending Transition to Duodenoscopes with Innovative Designs to Enhance Safety: DA Safety Communication*.[15] Within the communication, the FDA recommends hos-itals and endoscopy suites consider transition to duodenoscopes with disposable omponents, with the understanding that transition likely is difficult for many institu-ons and that there is not yet an approved disposable device or cap. In the same ommunication, the FDA advises against utilizing adenosine triphosphate (ATP) test trips to assess duodenoscope cleaning, because there currently are no legally mar-eted, FDA-approved ATP test strips for such purposes. Additional reminders reit-rate their prior recommendations of ensuring staff are meticulous in following eprocessing instructions, instituting a quality control program, and monitoring eprocessing when possible by duodenoscope sampling and culturing.

Iultisociety guidelines on reprocessing flexible gastrointestinal endoscopes: 2016 pdate

, multisociety guidelines, published in *Gastrointestinal Endoscopy* in February 2017, erved to update guidelines from the reprocessing guideline taskforce, first published a 2011.[2] This document aimed to update reprocessing recommendations for duode-oscopes and linear echoendoscopes. The guideline was supported by the ASGE, CG, AGA, SGNA, the Association for Professionals in Infection Control and Epidemi-logy, the American Society of Colon and Rectal Surgeons, the American Association or the Study of Liver Diseases, and the Society of American Gastrointestinal and ndoscopic Surgeons.

An initial recommendation is provided for comprehensive cleaning of all flexible en-oscopes with at least HLD as recommended by multiple professional organizations. he guideline includes the FDA supplemental guidance for reprocessing of duodeno-copes. Overall, the guideline recommends following FDA or manufacturers' reproc-ssing instructions for specific devices. Exceptions may be made if there are everal high-quality scientific studies supported by professional societies enhancing 1ose existing reprocessing techniques. The guideline provides 41 recommendations or endoscope reprocessing.

There are 9 category IA and 11 category IB recommendations within the guideline, /hich are "strongly recommended for implementation" (**Table 2**). Four additional duo-enoscope reprocessing methods are considered category II recommendations, ecause none is validated. It is suggested that each facility should consider FDA sug-ested additional modalities for duodenoscope reprocessing, including intermittent or er procedure culture surveillance, EtO gas sterilization, a second application of stan-ard HLD, and use of liquid chemical sterilant.

Table 2
Multisociety category IA and category IIB recommendations, 2016

Category IA recommendations

- All health care personnel within the endoscopy suite should be trained in standard infection precautions.
- Sterilization of any reusable accessories between uses is required (HLD alone is insufficient).
- HLD is required for any endoscope or accessory contacting a mucous membrane.
- New HLDs and machines specific to these agents need to be utilized with independent information accessible via the FDA Web site and must be FDA approved.
- Temperature and time for disinfecting can vary depending on type of HLD used; this must be followed according to FDA-approved labeling for the various disinfectants.
- After HLD, endoscope channels must be flushed with sterile or filtered water, followed by flush with 70%–90% alcohol (isopropyl or ethyl), and dried using filtered forced air.
- HLD liquid should be routinely tested daily, or more frequently if recommended by the manufacturer, to assure the active ingredient minimal concentration is maintained.
- Personnel reprocessing endoscopes must receive device specific training, and their competency must be assessed at completion of their training, annually, and anytime a breach is suspected. No temporary personnel should reprocess endoscopes unless competency has been achieved and tested.
- Any outbreak should trigger environmental sampling in accordance with standard investigation protocols.

Category IIB recommendations

- Precleaning should occur prior to HLD with wiping of the exterior of the endoscope with detergent and aspiration of detergent through all endoscope channels.
- Pressure and leak testing should be performed after each use and before reprocessing.
- Manual cleaning of the endoscope, including all channels, valves, detachable parts and connectors with brushes or cleaning devices specific to the endoscope model must be performed within manufacturer's designated timeline. All components/valves must be disconnected, and the entire scope and components should be immersed in detergent per manufacturer instructions, along with thorough flush and brush of all channels. Valves must be actuated repeatedly while cleaning.
- Enzymatic detergents should be discarded after each use.
- Specific HLDs used should be assured to be compatible with the particular endoscope cleaned.
- HLD can be performed using an AER or a manual process. Usage of AER is preferred and it must be compatible with specific endoscopes cleaned. Assure if an AER is used that all components can be reprocessed effectively. For example, the elevator wire channel in duodenoscopes usually must be manually reprocessed when using an AER.
- Attach and place the endoscope and components within the AER with approved connectors and according to manufacturer guidelines.
- Immersion of the endoscope and all components completely within HLD solution.
- HLD or sterilization to the water bottle and connecting tube (for irrigation and lens cleaning) should be completed daily, along with sterile water used to fill the bottle.
- HLD solution may be single or multiple use but must be discarded when reuse life is exhausted per manufacturer guidelines.
- Endoscope disinfection and use areas should be safe for patients and health care workers with proper ventilation, eyewash stations, and other protective precautions.

(continued on next page)

Table 2 (continued)	
	• Report any endoscopy related infection outbreaks (to institutional infection control, designated public health agency, the FDA; and to the manufacturer of the endoscope, disinfectant, and AER.

CDC categorization of recommendations: category 1A: strongly recommended for implementation and strongly supported by well-designed experimental, clinical, or epidemiologic studies; category 1B: strongly recommended for implementation and supported by some experimental, clinical, or epidemiologic studies and a strong theoretic rationale.

Within this guideline, there are issues that are considered to need further evaluation. The hang time of the endoscope after processing refers to the length of time an endoscope can be stored without use after reprocessing. Although vertical hanging of reprocessed endoscopes is advised, no specific recommendation is made regarding maximum hang time, because "the available data suggest that contamination during the appropriate storage intervals of 7 to 21 days is negligible."[2] This contrasts with the 2018 SGNA guideline recommending maximum storage of 7 days without reprocessing.[14] Recommended frequency of replacement of lens wash water, insufflation and suction tubing, in addition to water bottles and waste vacuum canisters, is not designated. The lack of appropriate data is cited. No recommendations are given regarding routine sampling and culture, with a request for further research before routine culturing or sampling is implemented. No recommendations are provided for endoscope longevity or AER reprocessing and the investigators note overall that the best methods for cleaning, sterilization, and/or disinfection still are not well understood.

In 2018, the ASGE Quality Assurance in Endoscopy Committee published updated guidelines for infection control.[16] Recommendations are similar to the 2016 multisociety guidelines. These include emphasizing the importance of manual cleaning and "consideration" of 1 or more additional steps advised by the FDA (double reprocessing cycles, duodenoscope culturing, or sterilization) if institutionally feasible. There is no recommendation of endoscope storage time before reuse, although the committee cites studies suggesting storage time ranging from 5 days to 21 days appear safe. Having qualified personnel, process validation, and quality assurance and assessing staff competency at least annually also are highlighted.

Standards of Infection Prevention in Reprocessing Flexible Gastrointestinal Endoscopes, Society of Gastroenterology Nurses and Associates (SGNA)

The SGNA supported the 2016 multisociety guidelines but also published a separate guideline in December 2018.[14] The 34-page guideline was prepared in 2018 by the SGNA board of directors and provided an update to the document first published in 1996 with subsequent revisions in 2000, 2005, 2007, 2008, 2011, 2012, 2015, and 2016. The guideline suggests following manufacturers' instructions for use and reprocessing of specific endoscopes, with emphasis and focus on improvement of the HLD process. Specifically, there is a focus on effective manual cleaning, good visual inspection, strengthening training of the reprocessing staff, monitoring timing and steps of endoscope use, and increasing reliability of HLD. Additional focus is on limiting cross-contamination or microbial growth, choice of disinfectant, and strict adherence and oversight to assure quality reprocessing. The guideline notes that further research is needed in regard to sterilization versus HLD of duodenoscopes before promoting sterilization.

The guideline mentions several factors that can impede effectiveness of HLD, including complex endoscope design features, such as an elevator channel; age of an endoscope, leading to internal surface damage; personnel factors, such as lack of knowledge and inadequate staff or training; reprocessing steps that are prone to human error; and reprocessing equipment malfunctions. The importance of having a multidisciplinary team involved in reprocessing and overview of safety is emphasized, including no temporary personnel allowed to clean instruments. The designated leadership must be able to oversee reprocessing effectiveness and safety, and adequate access for reprocessing personnel to required time and equipment must be provided. Appropriate quality assurance is important, including adequate documentation of endoscope use and reprocessing, along with intermittent audits to monitor all reprocessing steps. Any suspected breaches in reprocessing must be addressed by predetermined facility policies and procedures. As in the multisociety guidelines, a clean and safe reprocessing environment, inclusive of procedure rooms, is required.

The SGNA endoscope reprocessing protocol is organized into 9 main categories, including precleaning, leak testing, manual cleaning, rinse after cleaning, visual inspection, HLD (manual or automated), rinse after HLD, drying, and storage. In contrast to the multisociety guidelines, which largely refer to FDA and manufacturer instructions for step-by-step reprocessing details, the SGNA protocol provides specific, detailed, step-by-step instructions.

The precleaning phase occurs just after endoscope removal from the patient and involves wiping of the endoscope with a detergent-soaked cloth or sponge and flush/suction of all channels with detergent. Similar to the multisociety guidelines, leak testing is recommended according to manufacturers' guidelines after each use prior to immersion in reprocessing solution, with detailed mechanical (wet) leak testing instructions provided within the guidelines.

Manual cleaning also is endorsed by the SGNA prior to HLD, with a recommendation to follow the manufacturers' defined time constraints. The SGNA notes, "this is the most critical step in removing the microbial burden from an endoscope."[14] Thorough brushing of all channels, with particular attention to complex components, such as elevators, is required. A detailed 12-step process is defined to be completed with manufacturer-approved brushes for specific endoscopes, with extra steps for duodenoscope elevator channels per manufacturers' instructions. Similar to the multisociety guidelines, if the time constraint for manual cleaning is not met, manufacturer recommendations for delayed recleaning and reprocessing must be followed. The endoscope and all removable parts should be rinsed after manual cleaning to remove any residual detergent or debris with forced air used to flush water from any channels.

A visual inspection then is recommended, in concordance with the multisociety guidelines, which recommend visual inspection during all stages of handling and reprocessing. SGNA further recommends use of a camera or borescope for internal channel inspection if available. Any damaged endoscopes or imperfections noted need to be addressed because these may compromise reprocessing.

Next, HLD is recommended. HLD fluid is recommended to be tested and monitored strictly according to manufacturer instructions. Manual or AER HLD is deemed appropriate. Detailed instructions are provided for either manual or AER HLD, with the caveat that manual disinfection of elevator wire channel of duodenoscopes must be performed if an AER is used. AER manufacturer recommendations should be followed strictly and carefully. Additional considerations (but not recommendations or requirements) for duodenoscope reprocessing include microbiological culturing, repeat HLD, tO sterilization, and liquid chemical sterilization. Endoscopes that have completed processing should not sit for an extended period (such as overnight) within the ER. A thorough rinse of all surfaces, removal parts, and channels with clean water nould be performed after HLD.

Drying of the endoscope is of utmost importance, because inadequate drying has een implicated in prior endoscope infections, and retained moisture promotes biofilm ccumulation. Thorough drying is accomplished with flushing of 70% to 90% ethyl or opropyl alcohol, followed by drying via AER-delivered or manually delivered filtered r.

Storage consists of free vertical hanging in purpose-designed storage cabinets. rying cabinets under pressure or standard storage cabinets are both acceptable. he SGNA recommends a 7-day storage period hang time for reprocessed endoscopes, while recognizing that there is no consensus between professional organizations. The SGNA guideline recommends further research into detergent efficacy gainst biofilm, improvement in endoscope design, detailed reprocessing steps, efficient drying, water quality, and standardized quality monitoring.

ternational Guidelines

 contrast to their American counterparts, international endoscope reprocessing uidelines typically are much more detail-oriented and process-oriented. For instance, he United Kingdom guidelines for decontamination of flexible endoscopes are a technical tour de force, spanning 244 pages across 5 articles. The bulletin covers wide-anging topics, from design and installation of endoscope reprocessing units to validation testing methods according to international standards (ISO 15883-4). A compendium of various international guidelines is provided.

anada

he 2010 Public Health Agency of Canada (PHAC) Infection Prevention and Control iuideline (IPCG) provides a systematic summary of currently available literature for ndoscope reprocessing.[17] Approximately three-quarters of the recommendations 1/97) are assigned evidence grade II, meaning the statements are based on non–old standard evidence (ie, from case series). This is a reflection, however, of the ick of available randomized control trials; the investigators note, "[r]obust evidence pon which to formulate these guidelines is scarce...".

Like many international guidelines, the Canadian guidelines emphasize the crucial ole of adequate manual brushing. It is difficult to understate the importance of this tep, because insufficient brushing increases the risk of biofilm formation, which is ighly advantageous to bacterial survival during HLD and subsequent bacterial transmission to patients.

Appropriately, the IPCG recommends maximal drying (from alcohol flush to forced ir drying to ventilated cabinets) to reduce the likelihood of postprocessing bacterial roliferation. A 7-day maximum storage time is promulgated, which is in line with GNA guidelines.

In direct contrast to European/Australian guidelines, however, the Canadian (and IS) guidelines do not recommend routine microbiologic culture in the absence of n outbreak or an identified reprocessing error.

An entire subsection is devoted to the theoretic risk of endoscopic transmission of ariant Creutzfeldt-Jakob disease (CJD) in scenarios of possible lymphoid tissue contact (eg, ileal biopsies), although there has never been a documented case of endocopic transmission of classic CJD or variant CJD.

Australia

The third edition of the Australian guidelines, released in 2010, is a process-based document, detailing everything from frequency of emergency endoscope reprocessing (every 72 hours) to the frequency of cultures for both AER machines and endoscopes (every 1–3 months, depending on scenario) to the test method of ultrasonic cleaning machines.[18] In a prophetic observation, the Australian guidelines are not confident about the role of ATP in evaluation of reprocessing protocols, which the FDA (as discussed previously) also explicitly discouraged in the use for evaluating duodenoscope cleanliness. Again, the importance of scrupulous manual cleaning is repeatedly emphasized across the 63-page document.

In contrast to Canadian/British guidelines, Australian guidelines no longer require dedicated endoscopes for theoretic concerns of classic CJD transmission through endoscopy.

Europe

The 2017 guidelines from the European Society of Gastrointestinal Endoscopy (ESGE) focus particularly on expectations regarding the device manufacturer[19]—not only should reprocessing staff follow a clearly laid out and detailed manufacturer's instructions for use but also manufacturers are expected to release updated information whenever a device redesign reoccurs (likely in reference to the new generation of duodenoscopes with sealed elevator channels, wherein the O-rings were found to hinder effective HLD and be a potential reservoir for bacteria[20]). There is no discussion of CJD risk in the 2017 ESGE guidelines.

Meanwhile, the British Society of Gastroenterology (BSG),[21] out of necessity, continues to tailor recommendations to reduce the risk of theoretic endoscopic CJD transmission, including the avoidance of alcohol and glutaraldehyde because both are known to fix proteins. There is some leeway allowed for time from endoscope use to AER reprocessing (up to 3 hours) as long as the channels remain moist, to account the possibility of endoscope reprocessing rooms located at remote facilities. In contrast to the ESGE, the BSG guidelines do not advise routine microbiologic surveillance cultures.

Asia/International

The Chinese and International (World Endoscopy Organization [WEO]) guidelines are unique in their tailored focus to endoscopic reprocessing realities in a developing country.[22–24] Guidelines from the Chinese Society of Digestive Endoscopy (CSDE) for example, devote several subsections toward the pursuit of high-quality infection control, from room design to hand hygiene.[23] For instance, it is advised that clean and contaminated areas of an endoscope room should be separated, lest there be cross-contamination. Areas where advanced endoscopy procedures are performed (ie, use of elevator scopes) should be fitted with an AER "if conditions allow," perhaps in acknowledgment of potentially limited resources at various Chinese endoscopy units. The CSGE guidelines advise separating upper and lower endoscope AER machines, or at least separating wash times.

The 2011 WEO guidelines explicitly acknowledge infection control challenges in a developing world, either as a function of culture or limited resources.[24] Many of the recommendations are broken down into a cascade of options, depending on whether a location's resources are limited (for example, using potable water and soap at an absolute minimum for endoscope reprocessing), medium (for example, using new detergent for each procedure), or extensive (for example, AER use). A 2017 WEO update on hygiene in Asian and Middle East endoscopy units reinforces key concepts of hygiene in line with reprocessing guidelines from developed countries.[22] For instance, single-use accessories (eg, forceps) should not be used more than once.

Lastly, the 2019 World Gastroenterology Organisation (WGO) guidelines have a rather comprehensive focus on biofilm and carbapenem-resistant Enterobacteriaceae prevention, which are identified as potential threats in modern-day endoscopy laboratories.[22,25] For example, it is advised that sinks are upgraded with the latest best-practice designs to minimize spray and overflow of waste water, which has been shown in laboratory-controlled environments to allow dispersal of microorganisms as much as 3 meters away from the sink trap. Similarly, due to the increasingly complex nature of duodenoscope reprocessing, this guideline encourages readers to ask critically whether their unit's ERCP procedural volumes warrant continued service line offering.

SUMMARY

Duodenoscope infection transmission is an increasingly recognized problem in ERCP.[1] Existing guidelines and protocols provide recommendations for endoscope reprocessing, in addition to specific protocols and recommendations regarding sampling, culture, and optional supplemental steps in reprocessing for duodenoscopes.[10,12,13] The imperative aspect of all of the guidelines is to provide consistent high-quality manual cleaning, followed by HLD and proper storage. Individuals involved in reprocessing should be well trained and scrutinized at regular intervals to assure strict adherence to manufacturers' and institutional reprocessing instructions. Oversight and documentation of endoscope use, reprocessing, and the personnel involved are important. Optional further steps in reprocessing of duodenoscopes include sampling and culturing, additional HLD cycle, and sterilization with EtO gas or liquid chemical sterilant. In the United States, implementation of additional steps is still advisable based on the feasibility of individual institutions. This differs from Australian guidelines, which recommend culturing not only duodenoscopes but also AER on a routine basis.

The future of duodenoscopes and ERCPs will rely heavily on the recently published FDA recommendation for use of disposable duodenoscopes or duodenoscopes with disposable components. Pathogen contamination and transmission rates with these new technologies and equipment is entirely uncertain. On March 30, 2019, the ASGE Duodenoscope Infection Control Summit, with 60 leaders and experts in the field, met to discuss recent developments, epidemiologic impact of the issue, and gaps in the present strategies. Excellent communication and collaboration between facilities, societies, endoscope manufacturers, and regulatory bodies are necessary for continued reprocessing protocol development and proper implementation of new disposable-component technologies.

DISCLOSURE

The authors have nothing to disclose.

REFERENCES

1. Rahman MR, Perisetti A, Coman R, et al. Duodenoscope-associated infections: update on an emerging problem. Dig Dis Sci 2019;64(6):1409–18.

2. Petersen BT, Cohen J, Hambrick RD 3rd, et al. Multisociety guideline on reprocessing flexible GI endoscopes: 2016 update. Gastrointest Endosc 2017;85(2): 282–94.e1.

3. Higa JT, Gluck M, Ross AS. Duodenoscope-associated bacterial infections: a review and update. Curr Treat Options Gastroenterol 2016;14(2):185–93.

4. Kovaleva J, Peters FT, van der Mei HC, et al. Transmission of infection by flexible gastrointestinal endoscopy and bronchoscopy. Clin Microbiol Rev 2013;26(2): 231–54.

5. Schaefer MK, Jhung M, Dahl M, et al. Infection control assessment of ambulatory surgical centers. JAMA 2010;303(22):2273–9.

6. Epstein L, Hunter JC, Arwady MA, et al. New Delhi metallo-beta-lactamase-producing carbapenem-resistant Escherichia coli associated with exposure to duodenoscopes. JAMA 2014;312(14):1447–55.

7. Kola A, Piening B, Pape UF, et al. An outbreak of carbapenem-resistant OXA-48 - producing Klebsiella pneumonia associated to duodenoscopy. Antimicrob Resist Infect Control 2015;4:8.

8. Higa JT. Duodenoscope-related infections: overview and epidemiology. Tech Gastrointest Endosc 2019;21:1–5.

9. Inc. OA. Urgent Safety Notification. Important Updated Labeling Information: New Reprocessing Instructions for the Olympus TJF-Q180V Duodenoscope. 2015.

10. FDA. Supplemental measures to enhance duodenoscope reprocessing. FDA Safety Communications; 2015.

11. FDA. Reprocessing medical devices in health care settings: validation methods and labeling. Guidance for Industry and Food and Drug Administration Staff; 2015.

12. FDA/CDC/ASM. Duodenoscope Surveillance Sampling & Culturing. Reducing the Risks of Infection. 2018.

13. Herrin A, Loyola M, Bocian S, et al. Standards of infection prevention in reprocessing flexible gastrointestinal endoscopes. Gastroenterol Nurs 2016;39(5): 404–18.

14. Loyola MB, Babb E, Bocian S, et al. Standards of infection prevention in reprocessing of flexible gastrointestinal endoscopes. Society of Gastroenterology and Nurses Associates, Inc; 2018. p. 34.

15. FDA. The FDA is recommending transition to duodenoscopes with innovative designs to enhance safety. FDA Safety Communication; 2019.

16. Calderwood AH, Day LW, Muthusamy VR, et al. ASGE guideline for infection control during GI endoscopy. Gastrointest Endosc 2018;87(5):1167–79.

17. Canada PHAo. Infection Prevention and Control Guideline for Flexible Gastrointestinal Endosocpy and Flexible Bronchoscopy. 2010.

18. Taylor A, Jones D, Everts R, et al. Infection control in endoscopy. Gastroenterological Society of Australia; 2010.

19. Beilenhoff U, Biering H, Blum R, et al. Prevention of multidrug-resistant infections from contaminated duodenoscopes: position Statement of the European Society of Gastrointestinal Endoscopy (ESGE) and European Society of Gastroenterology Nurses and Associates (ESGENA). Endoscopy 2017;49(11):1098–106.

20. United States Senate. Health E, Labor, and Pensions Committee. Patty Murray. Preventable Tragedies: Superbugs and How Ineffective Monitoring of Medical Device Safety Fails Patients. 2016.

1. Working Party of the British Society of Gastroenterology Endoscopy Committee. BSG guidance for decontamination of equipment for gastrointestinal endoscopy. London: British Society of Gastroenterology; 2016.
2. Murdani A, Kumar A, Chiu HM, et al. WEO position statement on hygiene in digestive endoscopy: focus on endoscopy units in Asia and the Middle East. Dig Endosc 2017;29(1):3–15.
3. Chinese Society of Digestive Endoscopy. Consensus of experts on the safe operation of digestive endoscopy centers in China. J Dig Dis 2016;17(12):790–9.
4. Rey JF, Bjorkman D, Nelson D, et al. Endoscope disinfection - a resource-sensitive approach. World Gastroenterology Organisation/World Endoscopy Organization Global Guidelines; 2011.
5. Speer T, Alfa M, Cowen A, et al. Endoscope disinfection update: a guide to resource-sensitive reprocessing. World Gastroenterology Organisation Global Guidelines; 2019.

Statement of Ownership, Management, and Circulation
(All Periodicals Publications Except Requester Publications)

UNITED STATES POSTAL SERVICE®

1. Publication Title	2. Publication Number	3. Filing Date
GASTROINTESTINAL ENDOSCOPY CLINICS OF NORTH AMERICA	012 – 603	9/18/2020

4. Issue Frequency	5. Number of Issues Published Annually	6. Annual Subscription Price
JAN, APR, JUL, OCT	4	$359.00

7. Complete Mailing Address of Known Office of Publication (Not printer) (Street, city, county, state, and ZIP+4®)

ELSEVIER INC.
230 Park Avenue, Suite 800
New York, NY 10169

Contact Person: Malathi Samayan
Telephone (Include area code): 91-44-4299-4507

8. Complete Mailing Address of Headquarters or General Business Office of Publisher (Not printer)

ELSEVIER INC.
230 Park Avenue, Suite 800
New York, NY 10169

9. Full Names and Complete Mailing Addresses of Publisher, Editor, and Managing Editor (Do not leave blank)

Publisher (Name and complete mailing address)
DOLORES MELONI, ELSEVIER INC.
1600 JOHN F KENNEDY BLVD. SUITE 1800
PHILADELPHIA, PA 19103-2899

Editor (Name and complete mailing address)
KERRY HOLLAND, ELSEVIER INC.
1600 JOHN F KENNEDY BLVD. SUITE 1800
PHILADELPHIA, PA 19103-2899

Managing Editor (Name and complete mailing address)
PATRICK MANLEY, ELSEVIER INC.
1600 JOHN F KENNEDY BLVD. SUITE 1800
PHILADELPHIA, PA 19103-2899

10. Owner (Do not leave blank. If the publication is owned by a corporation, give the name and address of the corporation immediately followed by the names and addresses of all stockholders owning or holding 1 percent or more of the total amount of stock. If not owned by a corporation, give the names and addresses of the individual owners. If owned by a partnership or other unincorporated firm, give its name and address as well as those of each individual owner. If the publication is published by a nonprofit organization, give its name and address.)

Full Name	Complete Mailing Address
WHOLLY OWNED SUBSIDIARY OF REED/ELSEVIER, US HOLDINGS	1600 JOHN F KENNEDY BLVD. SUITE 1800 PHILADELPHIA, PA 19103-2899

11. Known Bondholders, Mortgagees, and Other Security Holders Owning or Holding 1 Percent or More of Total Amount of Bonds, Mortgages, or Other Securities. If none, check box ▶ ☐ None

Full Name	Complete Mailing Address
N/A	

12. Tax Status (For completion by nonprofit organizations authorized to mail at nonprofit rates) (Check one)
The purpose, function, and nonprofit status of this organization and the exempt status for federal income tax purposes:
☒ Has Not Changed During Preceding 12 Months
☐ Has Changed During Preceding 12 Months (Publisher must submit explanation of change with this statement)

PS Form **3526**, July 2014 [Page 1 of 4 (see instructions page 4)] PSN: 7530-01-000-9931 PRIVACY NOTICE: See our privacy policy on www.usps.com

---

13. Publication Title	14. Issue Date for Circulation Data Below
GASTROINTESTINAL ENDOSCOPY CLINICS OF NORTH AMERICA	JULY 2020

15. Extent and Nature of Circulation		Average No. Copies Each Issue During Preceding 12 Months	No. Copies of Single Issue Published Nearest to Filing Date
a. Total Number of Copies (Net press run)		138	121
b. Paid Circulation (By Mail and Outside the Mail)	(1) Mailed Outside-County Paid Subscriptions Stated on PS Form 3541 (Include paid distribution above nominal rate, advertiser's proof copies, and exchange copies)	57	47
	(2) Mailed In-County Paid Subscriptions Stated on PS Form 3541 (Include paid distribution above nominal rate, advertiser's proof copies, and exchange copies)	0	0
	(3) Paid Distribution Outside the Mails Including Sales Through Dealers and Carriers, Street Vendors, Counter Sales, and Other Paid Distribution Outside USPS®	25	25
	(4) Paid Distribution by Other Classes of Mail Through the USPS (e.g. First-Class Mail®)	0	0
c. Total Paid Distribution (Sum of 15b (1), (2), (3), and (4))	▶	82	72
d. Free or Nominal Rate Distribution (By Mail and Outside the Mail)	(1) Free or Nominal Rate Outside-County Copies Included on PS Form 3541	40	32
	(2) Free or Nominal Rate In-County Copies Included on PS Form 3541	0	0
	(3) Free or Nominal Rate Copies Mailed at Other Classes Through the USPS (e.g. First-Class Mail)	0	0
	(4) Free or Nominal Rate Distribution Outside the Mail (Carriers or other means)	0	0
e. Total Free or Nominal Rate Distribution (Sum of 15d (1), (2), (3) and (4))	▶	40	32
f. Total Distribution (Sum of 15c and 15e)	▶	122	104
g. Copies not Distributed (See Instructions to Publishers #4 (page #3))	▶	16	17
h. Total (Sum of 15f and g)	▶	138	121
i. Percent Paid (15c divided by 15f times 100)	▶	67.21%	69.23%

* If you are claiming electronic copies, go to line 16 on page 3. If you are not claiming electronic copies, skip to line 17 on page 3.

16. Electronic Copy Circulation	Average No. Copies Each Issue During Preceding 12 Months	No. Copies of Single Issue Published Nearest to Filing Date
a. Paid Electronic Copies	▶	
b. Total Paid Print Copies (Line 15c) + Paid Electronic Copies (Line 16a)	▶	
c. Total Print Distribution (Line 15f) + Paid Electronic Copies (Line 16a)	▶	
d. Percent Paid (Both Print & Electronic Copies) (16b divided by 16c × 100)	▶	

☒ I certify that 50% of all my distributed copies (electronic and print) are paid above a nominal price.

17. Publication of Statement of Ownership
☒ If the publication is a general publication, publication of this statement is required. Will be printed in the OCTOBER 2020 issue of this publication. ☐ Publication not required.

18. Signature and Title of Editor, Publisher, Business Manager, or Owner

Malathi Samayan Date 9/18/2020

Malathi Samayan - Distribution Controller

I certify that all information furnished on this form is true and complete. I understand that anyone who furnishes false or misleading information on this form or who omits material or information requested on the form may be subject to criminal sanctions (including fines and imprisonment) and/or civil sanctions (including civil penalties).

PS Form **3526**, July 2014 (Page 3 of 4) PRIVACY NOTICE: See our privacy policy on www.usps.com

Moving?

Make sure your subscription moves with you!

To notify us of your new address, find your **Clinics Account Number** (located on your mailing label above your name), and contact customer service at:

Email: journalscustomerservice-usa@elsevier.com

800-654-2452 (subscribers in the U.S. & Canada)
314-447-8871 (subscribers outside of the U.S. & Canada)

Fax number: 314-447-8029

Elsevier Health Sciences Division
Subscription Customer Service
3251 Riverport Lane
Maryland Heights, MO 63043

*To ensure uninterrupted delivery of your subscription, please notify us at least 4 weeks in advance of move.

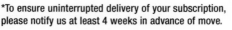
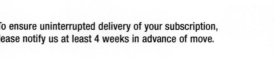